I Have Not

Seen My Family

In Over Ten Months

All immediate family members are desperate to see their loved ones on the Isle of Man.

The Manx Governments Ten month and counting Border ban on families is abusive. Immediate family ARE NOT visitors, they are family of residents, LET US IN!

To Manx Residents,

Allowing immediate family onto the island is less risky than allowing the 41,077 travelling residents that the Manx Government have allowed to leave and return. Don't let the Manx Government brain wash and lie to you.

How can any decent person say that the Manx can come to the UK and then return to IOM and self-isolate for 14 days. While immediate family are not given the same rights?

What if the UK had kept the Manx people from visiting their families in the UK and put a ban to stop the Manx for over 10 months coming to the UK? It would be a totally different story.

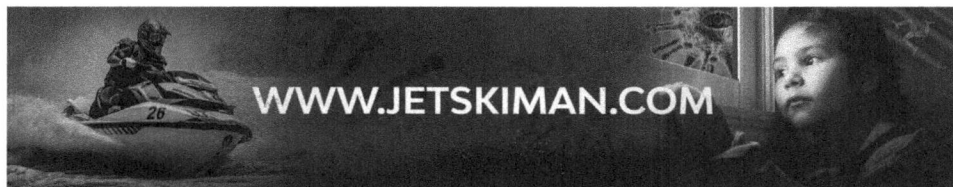

WWW.JETSKIMAN.COM

Contents

Disclaimer

The publisher and author would like to make it clear:

- Do not do what Dale did. In fact if you feel compelled to make a stand for justice, then we suggest that you speak to a legal advisor first.
- At no time are we asking or recommending that you do what Dale did or to break another countries laws. However, we do live in a world of democracy, and laws & legislation can be freely challenged. How you go about that is entirely your choice and your decision, but since we live in a world were law is forced upon you, then I would suggest that you take legal advice first before any action.
- The Isle of Man is subject to European and International laws and as such will be held fully accountable for its deprivation of immediate family's rights to visit their family on the Isle of Man
- It was reported that Dale could not swim and it was the first time he rode a Jet Ski. It is important that you do not put your life or any other person's life at risk (For example if Dale had got into trouble at sea, the emergency response team's lives could be in danger.)
- People do have a right to peaceful protest and to challenge unjust rules, regulations, laws and injustices. Don't let authorities dismiss you, you are the ones paying their wages.
- Freedom is a basic right and unjust Covid laws by some countries cannot be tolerated, as such every person has a right to justice and to challenge laws especially ones that keep families apart.
- Dale was not contacted at any time for his comments or views, nor do we know anything about Dale. As such the author and publisher want to make it clear that all information about Dale is purely in relation to that sea journey to the Isle of Man via research on the topic.

.Donations and Assistance

1. Fighting for Climate Justice
2. Finding missing Children and Adults
3. Mental Health & Suicide Prevention Awareness

To help me in my three causes: If you like what you read and are in a position to make a donation then you can do so by any of the following methods.

Methods of support:

1. Purchase the paperback version of this book.

Or
2. Purchase my book 'Missing in Paris' by Dave Smith on Amazon or other booksellers (My True story on finding a missing teenager in Paris)

Or
3. You can make a direct donation at:
https://www.paypal.me/ClimateCancer

Or
4. Become a climate activist **or** help find missing people, **or** become aware of mental health issues and how you can help others.

Dave is also available for book club tours and talks on "Climate Change," or "Adverse Childhood Experiences," Or "Suicide Awareness"

Dave is a Climate Reality Leader and does not charge any fees to make a Climate Reality presentation. Dave is proud to say that he was trained by Vice President Ali Gore and the Climate Reality Project team. Without activist the world would be in a worse state.

Dave Smith has asserted his right to be identified as the author of this work in accordance with the Copyright, Designs and Patients Act 1988. A CIP catalogue record for this book is available from the Irish, Scottish, Welsh and British Libraries.

Published (December 2020) © by Three Zombie Dogs, McLaughlin's Close, Derry, BT486SZ.

- Cover design by: Olivia Pro Design
- Breaking News Video: Jeffrey Hopkins and Lyrics by Dave Smith
- Twelve days of Christmas song: Music By Bethany and Lyrics by Dave Smith
- 2021 New Year message Video: Blue7trawberry
- Images by: Enrique Lopezgarre, Dimitris Vetsikas and Jorono [from Pixabay]
- Paperback ISBN: 9781912039050

Three Zombie Dogs are committed to ensuring that any printer adheres to sourcing their paper from responsible and sustainable sources and TZD plant trees via an approved programme for every book sold.

Go to http://www.saytrees.org and see how you can help

Dedication:

To EVERY person working within essential services. They are ALL ensuring that the rest of the population can remain safe. They are everyone's heroes. A special thanks to all shop staff, these people have been on the front line, dealing with thousands of people, face to face in an extreme close proximity on a daily basis and with no protective equipment. I believe that this was a shamble by the Governments not to provide these essential workers with protective equipment from day one. Even today some still don't have any protective equipment or clothing.

Practice Safe Distancing and wear a mask in public places, Keep the NHS safe from overloading, otherwise they will not be in a good position to help your loved one.

To everyone around the world

Young and old please stay safe. The health message has been clear; the older and more vulnerable you are, the more at risk you are from COVID and its new virus strain. However, the World Health Organisation has warned young people should not view themselves as "invincible". Some young people are dying, so please listen to the advice about locking down and keeping a safe social distance.

Authors Statement

I like many other immediate family members have been denied entry to visit our immediate family for almost TEN months from publication of this book.

That's TEN months removed from my life and is a direct breech of human rights. It is morally wrong and is disgusting beyond belief.

Immediate family are requesting the same rights as returning residents, and they will self-isolate on the IOM for the 14 days as is for returning residents. Immediate family can take a Covid test before departing and another test on their arrival in the Isle of Man.

We are not saying that the IOM should open its doors and allow everyone in. But we are asking that immediate family be given the same rights as returning residents.

Immediate family coming to the IOM pose no greater risk than that of returning residents. 41,077 Manx residents (49% of the population) travelled to and from the IOM between 1st April and 30th November.

The Manx public have been brainwashed and forced to be fearful of people who are not Manx residents. This is an abuse of Governmental power, it is small mindlessness and corruption to the core. Did the Manx hide when the rest of the world were battling it out to save humankind during the 1st and 2nd world war? So why are they creating double standards now by allowing their residents free travel but not allowing immediate family access?

European and International legislation has stated that closing borders for long periods is unlawful and morally wrong. They have further stated that Draconian restrictions should be systemically rejected. Covid qualifies as a disease with epidemic potential, nevertheless any restrictions have to comply with the principal of proportionality. As such the Isle of Man are GUILTY of breaking EU and UN human rights, family Justice and the right of free movement. No other country in the world has stopped immediate family entry for as long as the Manx Government have done.

Jet Ski Man

"They'll never take our Freedom"

Exiting a Pandemic

Dale did what was necessary to be with the love of his life.

Would you have done the same?

Would you be willing to undertake peaceful and legal protests at airports and sea terminals departing/arriving to/from the Isle of Man to raise International awareness?

Dale's Girlfriend pleads with the Manx Government to set him free in time for Christmas. Dale is released, but is deported to Scotland just in time to spend Christmas with his own children, but sadly not on the Isle of Man.

Dale, your mission if you choose to accept it:

- Jet Ski to the Isle of Man and break through the Manx Governments inconsiderate and illegitimate ban of not allowing immediate family entry to the island.

- Do not raise suspicion, and you are to do the "Mr Bean" method of getting to Ramsey. Jet Ski for five hours and not the forty minutes you had previously planned to thwart them from your trail.

- You must not infect the Manx residents with your super-duper infecting genes that returning resident don't have. So do not take buses or Taxis, but walk 25 km to Douglas. And make sure you walk like a hero, that's if your 3 legs will allow you to do that. Though one leg might be a bit shrivelled from the sea sprays and the coldness?

- When you arrive in Douglas, go straight to this address [xxx], knock twice, wait three seconds, then knock once more on Jessica's Christmas door, and she will have a password for you.

- Your cover will be that of the artist "Young Thug" when Jessica opens the door and sees her hero standing there, she will alluringly sing that secret password to you. Then and only then will you know it's safe to enter her doorway to heaven.

- Remember to wear protection at all times. Jessica's password: *"She like, Wet me like a jet-ski."*

- Good luck. And remember, stay low, those Manx Spies are out there lurking in every dark and bright corner. They can seek out "COME-OVERS" with one twitch of an R......A......T's nose, unless of course you are rich and affluent.

- This tape will self-destruct in five seconds, unless you hit the replay button …☺

You have to concede that there was something sexy and adventurous in what Dale did just to be by his girlfriend's side or he could have been an utter nutter? But there is a flip side to every coin and it tells a different side of the same story.

The Manx Government and their prosecutors will have you believe their Covid laws are valid and will be enforced. But why should the Dale's or any other person who has immediate family on the Isle of Man respect or indeed obey Manx laws? Especially when the Manx law and Government does not respect the basic international right of immediate family to be given access to visit their families?

The last time someone imposed such rules on a nation was Hitler and look what happened. Hitler believed his laws were "just, legal and reasonable," and we all know that was furthest from the truth. The Manx Government in their selfishness and blinkered sight believe that they have the right to ban immediate family from visiting their immediate family on the Isle of Man for ten months and counting.

What Dale did was not uncommon but nevertheless such a journey does pose a risk to the rider's life. Did Dale carry spare fuel with him or was it a free for all dash to be with the love of his life?

In 2002 Count Alvaro de Marichalar took four months to cross the Atlantic Ocean to Miami in a jet ski. He spend 12 hours per day standing up on his jet ski just to avoid injury to his spine. The count had something Dale did not have and that was a supply ship following him to provide food, water and security.

Another brave Jet Skier was Risto Piispa from Finland who undertook an epic 3704 km Jet Ski journey that had no support ships for his self-sacrificing act of getting into the Guinness book of records just to raise money for charity.

But riding a Jet Ski is not always exciting and sexy, there have been many fatalities over the years. Jet Skiing like some other sports, does carry an element of high risk. But risk is also an element of human growth and development, and that forms part of a person's developing psyche. With these inconsiderate laws that the Manx Government have deployed, especially during Covid, instigates a need of unlawful risk taking in order to achieve what is your birth right claim. A person's birth-right claim is greater, and overshadows, and is certainly above any manmade law.

Your birth right is of human connection, your birth right is being with your immediate family. Though in times of emergencies and pandemics that might not always be immediately possible. However, two weeks to six weeks is an acceptable time to spend apart or at least until corrective measures to address this separation is found and implemented. But over nine months is not acceptable by any standards, and especially when the same Manx Government allows 49% of its population to travel back and forth. What Dale did was understandable and justification.

The fact that the Manx Government department of health has not forced the Governments hand in addressing the psychological, emotional and physical needs of its resident's immediate families is a further sign of distrust in a Government that stinks of wealth before Health.

Twelve Days of Christmas Song (Manx Government version)
Music by Bethany, Lyrics by Dave Smith

I have been corresponding with the Isle of Man Government for several months and they will not budge on allowing any immediate and essential family members onto the Island, unless your loved one is dying or dead. Yet they allowed over 41,077 residents (49% of their population) to travel to and from the UK.

Immediate family wanting to come to the Isle of Man and self-isolate pose no greater risk than the 41,077 other residents who have travelled.

I want to apologise, I may be quite repetitive in my use of certain terms etc. This is only because they have a huge bearing in the counter claim that the Manx Government are actually doing a lockdown. They are not! They are misusing the generosity of other countries that allow Manx residents to travel while not allowing one immediate family access to the Isle of Man.

Please Tweet: #manxdoublestandards

I could have understood the Manx Governments stance not to let anyone onto the island via fear of the 75 million people infected around the world. However, this cannot be the case as they are not that fearful to have let 41,077 residents travel to and from the Island during 1st April 2020 and 30th November 2020. That's equivalent to 49% of the Manx population. As such they have removed any claim to protecting their residents via any lockdown concept that they have.

There really is no lockdown in the Isle of Man if they have allowed almost 50% of their residents to travel. And at the very least immediate family should be allowed to visit under the same rules as returning residents. Nine months and counting and the Manx Government have denied immediate family access to their families, this is what you would term International Human Rights Treason.

Active Cases

(Number of Infected People)

Currently Infected

The above graph shows that the number of cases in the Isle of Man are very low and in some instances they are reported as being non-existent. This low infection rate was primarily down to the lack of infected international travellers arriving to the Isle of Man prior to their lockdown in March 2020, as such the virus transmission rate was quite low within the Manx population. But the Manx Government have demonstrated that with 41,077 residents travelling and many breaking self-isolation rules they have still managed to keep numbers low. So why can't they let immediate family onto the Island while following the same self-isolation rules as returning and travelling residents?

In the correspondence section of this book you will notice that I have been accused of abusive comments. I vehemently deny this and reiterate that the only people being abusive are the Manx Government on their double standards and total lack of consideration for the health and wellbeing of immediate family of Manx residents.   Yes, I can claim to be guilty of being excessive and passionate with regards to my campaign to get justice for all of the islands resident's immediate family members from a tyranny of a Manx Government.

I would also like to point out that the American President Donald Trump called CNN reporters "Dumb Bastard's." Trump also called Beto O'Rourke a "poor bastard, a poor pathetic guy." Even more controversial is a band called "Kunt" whose song went straight into the UK charts. Their song is called "Boris Johnson is a F****** C***"

I did not call the Manx Government "Dumb Bastards or Poor Pathetic Bastards." Nor did I call the Manx Health Minister David Ashford or the Manx Chief Minister Howard Quayle a F****** C***. What I did say and I backed my claim up with a quotation from Colin's dictionary, "that they were Scumbags." However, I do regret lowering myself to use this word to describe the actions of a Manx Government who cares little for everyone in the world apart from themselves. But in reality the word that I used or the words used by Donald Trump or the punk band Kunt go nowhere near enough to describe what the Manx Government really are. How a Government can do what they have done is pathetic, cruel and a rogue and disgraceful nation.

Dale's act of Justice and release from his mental health anguishes of not being with his girlfriend manifested into a heroic and dangerous sea adventure of crossing the Irish Sea to be with his girlfriend. Which I do not recommend any person to do!

I'm writing this section of Jet Ski Man as a release from my mental health and frustration caused by being denied access to my immediate family for nearly ten months. I want the world to know and I want the world to act. Dale's adventure and my protest writing are symbolic and were actioned by an uncaring and unscrupulous Manx Government.

Number of residents, new residents and new workers travelling 'on and off' the Isle of Man. Yet not one immediate family allowed entry except if they are arriving for the dead or their dying family members.

Date (2020)	By Boat	By Plane
April	375	294
May	643	505
June	1,027	1,019
July	2,445	2,795
August	4,538	7,412
September	4,570	5,239
October	2,715	3,385
November	1,886	2,229
Totals	18,199	22878
Overall Total	**41,077**	

Source of above: From the Isle of Man Government passenger arrivals.

Jet Ski Man

Donald Trump is the outgoing president of the United States of America and he made the following remark during his time in office:

"That makes me smart. Obeying the rules is for suckers and chumps."

So if this is true for an influential president, a billionaire, a person in an immense position of power and authority. Then why should the people of the UK obey the UK's crown dependency of the IOM's restrictions of not allowing immediate family access to their families on the IOM? The Manx Governments authoritarian and draconian pandemic measures are a display of unethical behaviour, and all done while the Manx Government allowed 49% of its own residents to travel freely. Without giving immediate family the same access rights as returning Manx residents.

Why should the residents of the UK allow this to happen when it's their tax money that is allowing the Isle of Man Government to continue to feed its wealthy?

Dale in his adventure of justice to be with his loved one, literally took the advice of a world leader and disobeyed the Manx Government's unethical Covid rules.

Did twenty eight year old Jet Ski Man Dale McLaughlan have a mental health issue when he risked his own life battling the choppy Irish Sea that has taken many a Manx fisherman's life to the ocean bed? His natural born instinct was to get to his loved one in the Isle of Man.

After this horrific sea journey that took nearly five hours, he then had to walk 25 km from Ramsey to Douglas which would have taken at least five more hours. The look on his girlfriend's face when he finally knocked on her door would have been priceless. Amazing stuff, a true hero and a justice activist fighting for the natural right to visit immediate family.

A human's basic natural instinct and right to be with one's family will always prevail over any Government's law. Every person born has that natural right, no one can take that away from you, and it is the basic right to human freedom, true equality and equal rights.

Borders are not a true entity of our existence as can be witnessed within climate change. Pollution from the USA or elsewhere affect us all regardless of where we live in the world. As such we cannot allow a countries borders to sustain a pathway to another pandemic, especially not the soon to be critical climate change pandemic that threatens our very existence. Governments need to ban fossil fuel mining and production with immediate effect and activist need to ensure that no country exercises any right to mine or continue to mine fossil fuels.

Back to the story after my climate rant. Was Dale a love struck romantic that desperately wanted to be at the side of his girlfriend that he missed so dearly? Never mind posting flowers or sending a box of chocolates. You can be your girlfriend's/boyfriend's real life action hero. Sweep her/him off their feet and into your heart by a heroism beyond believe or was it sheer foolishness on Dale's part?

It was further amusing when a local Manx business used this opportunity to advertise its delivery options, "let us send flowers or chocolates, rather than you undertaking this epic journey yourself." But sadly this business was clearly missing the point, it's been nine months since any immediate family has been allowed onto the Isle of Man. Therefore, the need to take action into a person's own hands becomes a necessity and a basic right and Manx law cannot be allowed to halt this.

Either way Dale was gallant to take on the Manx Government's draconian stance in not allowing immediate family onto the Island.

Belonging, closeness, touch and sex are some of the basic and natural human instincts and the ultimate right of every human being or indeed any creature on earth. This desire to be with your loved ones is stronger than a Government who denies these basic rights for immediate family. And to think Dale was only apart from his girlfriend for three months. The rest of us it's been nine months so far.

Psychologists and researchers throughout the world have been crystal clear in their research. For wellbeing and good mental health to exist, then physical and emotional contact with peers and immediate families is a pre-requisite. This basic human need and right is above any Governments attempt to keep family apart and especially apart for over nine months. At a bare minimum you would have thought that the advisors to the Manx MHK on Health would have made this matter clear.

The small and narrow mindlessness of the current Manx Government is astonishingly naïve, when they believe that they can get away with family separation for so long and by creating an unjust and 100% unethical border rule begs believe. To use the words of Donald Trump, **"Obeying the Manx Government rules are for suckers and chumps."**

The Manx Government's border restriction rule as applied to immediate family is unjust, corrupt, breaks international human rights and will not be tolerated. May the Heroic and justice seeking Dale's of this world continue to rise up, and flourish until the tyranny of a Manx Government is squashed.

No Government should be allowed to remove human basic needs, if it does then it has removed the natural right of each individual human to justice and when a Government refutes an individual justice, then they have removed a person's right to human justice. As such an individual has the right to take justice into their own hands, which Dale did. And for that he deserves good old fashioned pat on the back and a standing ovation from every person who believes in freedom and justice.

Just worth noting when I talk about justice and freedom that does not imply that any person has a right to put another person in danger. And by that I mean, people do need to self-isolate, people do need to protect each other from spreading the Covid virus, by social distancing, wearing masks etc., until we have Covid under control. But stopping immediate family from entry for over nine months is refuting freedom and human rights.

Justice is not reserved for a collectivism such as a Government. Justice is the basic right of each individual and sits high above any Government or legal system.

But the problem with justice is that it has become a commodity, and that does not serve the poor well. For example the best justice can be purchased by the rich or affluent. Dale did not have any money to purchase the legal services that the rich on the Island could afford. He was handed a court appointed legal defence. As such justice is not equal and fair to all people. If you are rich you get a better legal team. In many cases a person is denied access to justice because they don't have enough money to pay for a legal defence or for litigation against an abuser. However, in some cases they can get legal aid.

If law is forced upon you, then it should be fair and equal and not dependant on how much money you can afford to pay for the best top notch lawyers. This again is an injustice. Perhaps if Dale could have afforded to pay for the most expensive attorney on the island then just perhaps he may have got away from any sentencing with a telling off?

Dale has set a precedent for all the lovers on the Island and beyond. Now regardless of what you do for your girlfriend/boyfriend it will never be able to match what Dale did for his girlfriend. Woman/men on the Island will want more than what they have been traditionally used to, *"I'm off to the pub now, gal, you want me to bring you back some Manx kippers? This won't cut it anymore"*

Did Jet Ski Man have a right to do what he did? The answer to that question will depend on the mind-set of who you ask.

- According to the IOM Government he broke Manx Law.

- If you ask his girlfriend then she would say yes he does have a right

- If you ask me then I too approve, I just wished I was younger and able to do what he did.

- What do you think? _____

I fully agree with what Dale has done, and I believe he had every moral right and true justice to do what he did. I also think that it was not veracious on how the Manx Government backed Dale into a corner and forced him into action which ultimately put his life at risk.

Dale also made one fatal mistake, he went out to a night club with his girlfriend, and as such he could have put others at risk in the event that he was carrying Covid. Therefore, his lack of immediate respect for others was wrong. Did he deserve the 4 weeks in jail? Based on the facts I don't think he deserved a jail sentence at all. The reasons being

- Anyone who plans or does something so dangerous to his life must be showing severe signs of frustration which in turn affects a person's mental health's reasoning capacity. He should have received counselling and not within a prison setting.

- Dale took a Covid test that showed he was negative and did not come into contact with any other person before he departed the shores of bonnie Scotland. As such he was just as healthy and Covid free as any other Manx resident. By doing this he demonstrated that he was caring and that he did not want to hurt anyone else. As such I think that the Manx justice in this case was abusive and not contingent with a person suffering from a bout of mental health issues brought on by an inadequate Manx Covid border legislation. The rule of law in this case was inconsiderate and did not reflect appropriate justice.

However, I do believe that the self-isolation requirements imposed by the Manx Government is a fair and reasonable request for anyone arriving on the island to uphold.

It was interesting that it was a Scottish man who did this, as in the historical past the Scottish would be fighting for their freedom and justice from the oppressor. And I suppose in a way the devolved nations are still fighting for their freedom.

In the words from Brave Heart I say this to the heartless, abusive and oppressor that call themselves a Manx Government.

"They may take our lives, but they'll never take our freedom"

The three legs of Isle of Man stands for "Quocunque Jeceris Stabit" literally translates to "Whithersoever you throw it, it will stand."

Well Dale certainly threw himself at it, unfortunately it did not stand and he was jailed before being deported just before Christmas Day 2020 back to Scotland from an island that is a crown dependence of the UK.

The problem is the Isle of Man Government get away with injustice way too much. For example, a UK citizen needs to apply for a permit to work on the IOM, yet a Manx person does not need a permit to come work in the UK. So with that in mind it's no surprise that the Manx Government believe that they can allow 41,077 of its residents to travel during Covid and not have to let one immediate family member entry, and they try to justify their action by saying that Manx residents can travel to UK to see their family. Its crap and it stinks and it needs changed.

Dale was send off the Island after he finished his work, he was turned down in his previous applications to re-enter the IOM. Simply because he does not have the wealth to purchase a home on the island. That's what you term "use and abuse and then discard." This mentality is the norm for the Manx Government.

I and all the other immediate families pay taxes to the UK and we are yet further penalised by a Manx Government that is doing nothing to allow immediate family the same rights as any of the 41,077 other travelling residents that enter the UK. This is an absolute sham and disgrace that a Manx Government should be allowed to get away with. No wonder people like Dale have taken the law into their own hands.

The Manx Government have broken basic human rights, they could have put protective measures in place to allow immediate family access but they were to short sighted. The Manx Government do not have common sense or the experience to handle a pandemic effectively for the good of ALL concerned.

But what is sad the most: The Manx Government are useless captains that would say fuck you to the few who are struggling to get onto that life raft. The Manx Government are taking the stance of "me, me, me," Disgusting and downright degrading.

To the Manx Government you are an utter disgrace to humanity, your inconsideration and sheer neglect of your international duties towards humanity and justice is non-existent and in a time of a global pandemic instead of sticking together you have become egocentric and uncaring to your immediate family obligations, and also that of the world. The Manx Government represents a cancer of intolerance, and like all cancer this must be cut out.

The Sun newspaper reported that Dale could not even swim and had very little fuel left. It was further mentioned that the residents of the Isle of Man think he is "hero and a legend" for what he did. But obviously the tyranny of a Manx Government and their legal system thought otherwise.

When someone goes to these extremes it makes one think, it stirs the heart and makes you revisit why a person who risks his own life has to do so in the first place?

In my endeavours to get to the island to see my sons and grandchildren, I have thought of doing many things including parachuting into the Isle of Man to gain international attention and help in my plight for immediate family justice. But what Dale did was real, it was heroic and careless at the same time.

I can't get over the love that he demonstrated when he was willing to risk his own life battling seas that could turn perilous in seconds.

His girlfriend must be so proud and mad at him at the same time. We must ALL stand in solidarity and fight this demon of a tyrant that hides under an umbrella of being called the Manx Government, a Government who care nothing about immediate family and their resident's emotional and physical needs.

Dale is a modern day hero, the Robin Hood who stole a moment of justice back from Manx Governmental oppressors. Dale gave that moment of hope back to families that have not been given access for over nine months, while he cemented his love for his girlfriend. The world needs more like him

They say that love conquers all. Love brings us together, love can heal and destroy us. And love for immediate family is seriously lacking from the Manx Government.

Thompson et al. (2018) argued that, *"The Science is clear: Separating Families has Long-term Damaging Psychological and Health Consequences for Children, Families, and Communities."*

Yet the Health Minister David Ashcroft's reply to me makes it crystal clear that the Manx Government do not care. Moreover, further proof that they don't care is the fact that they have allowed 41,077 (49%) to travel without letting one immediate family member onto the island is

100% proof. For due diligence, I would like to point out that they do let immediate family onto the island when their family member is about to die or has died. I think Donald Trump would have said? "Sick B……." about that.

How any of these cabinet ministers and legal representatives can go home at night and look into the eyes of their loved ones while still believing that their stance is right, begs belief. How they can sleep at night knowing all too well that immediate family are in emotional turmoil and distraught at the Manx Governments so far nine month ban on letting immediate family onto the island is totally abusive and disgraceful.

The Manx Government's stance is sick, disgusting, inhuman, idiotic and breeches the rights and freedoms of a families basic needs. No other country in the world has banned immediate family for over nine months from visiting their loved ones.

I'm not the only one accusing the Manx Government of being tyrants. The Guardian newspaper has previously reported that the Isle of Man has been accused of 'authoritarian' lockdown measures and being inhumane in the way they have carried out their justice in this matter.

What is astonish is the fact that the International community have done very little to readdress this injustice. Are the Manx Government getting away with tyranny because they represent the rich and the affluent of the world and that they hold the hidden money of many Politian's and other people wishing to avoid paying their taxes?

Another aspect is that the UK is subsidising the rich and affluent via the Manx Government. As outlined in this statement by Dame Margaret Hodge in 2017:

"Without our subsidy, the Isle of Man could not afford to have a zero rate of corporation tax and could not function as a tax haven. The Isle of Man is well and truly a UK tax haven. Far from being at the

head of the fight against tax avoidance and evasion, and money laundering, we are at the heart of the evil conspiracy involving advisers, the super-rich, global corporations and Governments. We are aiding and abetting the very few wealthiest and most powerful in our society to keep their wealth secret and avoid paying their fair share of tax."

And that my readers is what you call scumbag tactics of a Government hell bend on being selfish, uncaring and who are in reality a disgrace to the ordinary decent Manx person.

The Manx Government have played their uncaring card very well, while they do not allow immediate family onto the Isle of Man they allowed 41,077 residents, that's 49% of their population to travel between 1st April 2020 and 30th November 2020. This is a massive kick in the teeth to its neighbours Scotland, North of Ireland, Ireland, Wales and England. Why should the UK and Irish Governments put up with these double standards? We are all tax payers, why should we allow the Manx to travel to our country when we can't travel to theirs?

The United Nationals needs to address this matter. What the Manx Government are doing is treacherous and beyond belief. So to Dale, well done man! You're an inspiration and a welcome breeze to a Government that stinks of corruption and cares not one ounce for the international community apart from what it can screw out of them.

My local MP has written on my behalf to the Secretary of State for Foreign, Commonwealth and Development Affairs to address the double standards that the Manx Government are displaying in regards to immediate family. [At the time of going to print I have not received a reply.]

Dale, you are the main actor in a true romantic movie that is actually real life. You play the part of Romeo and your girlfriend is Juliette. And of course the Manx Government are the evil people playing the primary antagonists role of being the Capulet and Montague families. It is sad to say this but people and nations around the world will grow to despise the Manx Governments massive breach in human rights.

I and many others gave the Manx Government the chance to mend their outrageous ways, we gave them solutions to fix this problem in a way that would ensure the continued safety of Manx residents. But the Manx Government would rather use and abuse its residents and the international community including that of the emotional and physical wellbeing of immediate family that are desperate to see their families.

In this special edition of "Exiting a Pandemic" you have witnessed the International injustices that the Isle of Man Government have committed. Moreover, they have dishonestly brain washed their residents into a mind-set that "non-residents arriving on the island will infect them." Yet the IOM Government have allowed over 41,077 Manx residents to travel to and from the UK from the sea and air terminals of the Isle of Man.[Arrival/departure sources: Isle of Man Government statistics, 1st April 2020 to 30th November 2020]

Can you honestly say or believe that immediate family members self-isolating on the Isle of Man possess a great health risk than the 41,077 travelling Manx people? I think not.

Definition of Immediate Family: Mothers, Daughters, Sisters, girlfriends, Fathers, Sons, Brothers and boyfriends.

As such it would be possible and morally correct to amend Manx Government Covid landing legislation to permit immediate family entry. Moreover, immediate family's self-isolation could be undertaken at special or fixed "self-isolation accommodation" on the Island, thus giving a needed boost to the Manx tourist accommodation and economy. Furthermore, the management of ensuring that immediate family visitors maintain their self-isolation would be far easier than what exists for any returning resident.

I know for a fact that quite a lot of returning Manx residents do not effectively self-isolate. Therefore, it is more than likely if an outbreak of Covid did resurface on the Isle of Man then it would more than likely have been introduced by some of the 41,077 travel residents.

As you can see there are many viable options for the Manx Government to allow at the very least immediate family access.

It is not morally correct, and it's breaking the United Nations charter on human rights when family are denied contact with their siblings on the Isle of Man. The Manx Government have denied immediate family access for nine months and counting, no other country in the world has done this terrible and immoral deed. They have totally discarded international and basic rights of a human to be in contact with immediate family, which in its self is disgusting, immoral and abusive.

The Manx Government have ensured that the Isle of Man will be documented in history as one of the least caring nations in the world. They will go down in history as the captains of a sinking ship that put themselves first and got into lifeboats while allowing all of their immediate family and neighbours to perish. Disgusting and immoral, but in reality what would you expect from a Government that thrives as an offshore tax haven protecting the rich and the affluent. All while the poor on the island have to suffer. The rich and affluent moving to the Isle of Man may have provided some jobs to the locals, but they have also pushed up property prices and the majority of residents cannot afford this. But hey that's another story that could fill another book. But it does display how immoral the Manx Government can be.

Guernsey Air Bridge

Who do you think travelled when the Guernsey air bridge was there? Certainly not the average Manx resident. I myself thought about flying to Guernsey, self-isolating there for two weeks and then travelling to the Isle of Man. But the financial cost was too great. But open your minds and think about that situation for one second, now step out of your brainwashed shoes and see the reality of this situation?

Please indulge me.

Guernsey were allowing any tom, dick and harry to arrive on its island as long as they self-isolated for 14 days on their arrival.

So, I would have been able to visit the Isle of Man legally with self-isolating in Guernsey for 14 days, then getting a flight to the Isle of Man. Have you grasped this fact so far?

So, is the Isle of Man Government not capable of allowing self-isolation on their shores for immediate family? Guernsey is a smaller island than Isle of Man, yet they allowed anyone entry. Is the current Manx cabinet and MHK's not educated or do they not possess the skills to do what the Guernsey Government did but better, thus ensuring Covid stayed at bay?

And remember the air bridge was in place while Guernsey were allowing anyone onto their island. In correspondence I sent to the Isle of Man's chief minister, I pointed out that the Isle of Man should at the very least allow immediate family entry to IOM. I also notified him that there was an immediate risk of Covid infection as Guernsey were allowing anyone onto the island and not just immediate family. To which I can sadly say I was right, Guernsey suffered an increase in Covid cases which resulted in the air bridge being removed.

This however, does not suggest that the Manx Government stance in not allowing immediate family access was correct. What occurred in Guernsey could have happened and still could in the Isle of Man. And any infection would mostly likely arise from one or a few of the 41,077 travelling residents, or new residents or people moving to a new home in the IOM.

However, I would add that the Guernsey Covid increase was attributed directly down to an incorrect self-isolation policy for its own returning residents and holiday makers. Please also note that while the air bridge was in affect between IOM and Guernsey, Guernsey were allowing family, business people and holiday makers to go to Guernsey. And remember that the Manx Government never allowed even one immediate family member access to the IOM, while allowing 41,077 people to travel, this highlights a huge lack of morality of this atrocious Manx Government.

I would further suggest to the Manx people that your only way out of this international mess and regain any International dignity or self-respect will be to use your vote at the next election. Do not vote for any of the existing MHK's, in fact stand for election yourselves, to get justice you must first remove the oppressors. The current Manx Government have failed the families of residents miserably. They have also failed the Manx people who struggle to be able to purchase and build a home for their own families.

Use Your

Vote Wisely

One of Many possible solutions to allow immediate family to visit

Q1) how can the Manx Government ensure an effective self-isolation policy?

Isle of Man relies on a strong tourist trade. It would be relatively easy to get local accommodation businesses on board and certain establishments could be ear market for strict self-isolation. Arriving immediate family etc. would stay in accommodation units that are held for families going into self-isolation on their arrival.

Q2) how would you manage peoples arrivals on different dates and where would they go?

First you have to remember that currently on the IOM anyone arriving on the island needs to have a pre-approved landing document. So the Government know how many are arriving as per their authorisation: Suggestion, have different accommodations for different weeks of landing. For example 30 people arrive week 1, they go the ABC hotel. Week 2 arrivals go to DEF Hotel and so forth, after 2 weeks that accommodation is freed up and can take week 3's arrivals, you catch the concept? Plus it is easier to manage and to ensure that people do self-isolate. Additional accommodation can be sought if numbers increase, plus there would be a control in place.

[Number of self-isolating beds available vs numbers destined to arrive]

For all returning residents, they go to their home and self-isolate together with a massive sign to be erected on their front door or lawn, "self-isolation in progress," that way police or neighbours can check plus locals know that this household is supposed to be self-isolating.

Testing is another possible concept used in conjunction with that of above. A Covid test to be undertaken prior to departure to the IOM. Then on arrival visitors and residents are retested as they go into self-isolation. That would highlight any possible problems for all that are self-isolating and would mitigate any doubt or problems.

My recommendations above are only a few but are totally manageable and flexible, they are food for thought towards a better way of mitigating possible Covid infections while allowing immediate family to travel to IOM. And it would make the Isle of Man even safer.

If you consider the fact that over 41,077 residents have travelled back and forth then there is an imminent risk that Covid infections could increase on the Isle of Man in the future. And the Manx news has many stories of residents and new workers not self-isolating. Moreover, if the Manx Government were to initiate my suggestions then they would actually protect Manx residents from returning residents who don't take self-isolation to seriously.

Due to Covid, the future landscape on a global bases has changed and as such Governments need to be able to transition to allow some sort of normality. But, doing what the Manx Government have done by banning all immediate family and others while allowing 41,077 Manx residents to travel is not a sustainable or a realistic way of life for anyone. The Manx Government have abused their power, they are supposed to be the carer of their residents, but their lack of true vision has blinded them to the true reality and that reality is people need their immediate families.

And as Dale has demonstrated romantic love or platonic love or family love conquers all else and especially the laws and legal system of a Manx Government that is hell bend on denying the international and basic rights of humanity.

To Dale, I would like to say a massive thank you, your youth and keenness to seek out justice is an inspiration to every vulnerable person in the world. The Manx Government have taken advantage of the vulnerable and their families.

To the residents of the Isle of Man, please do not vote these MHK's back into power. Take it upon yourself to do the right thing and stand for election as an MHK yourself. Stands for equality, justice and a Politian that will push for change to halt Climate Cancer.

To the Manx Government, you still have time to make amends, first open your borders so that immediate family members have the same rights as returning residents, or new residents, or people moving to live on the Island. Second pay compensation to the immediate family members that you have emotionally affected as per correspondence that I have send you.

No self-respecting person could vote for the current MHK's knowing that they were against immediate family getting access to IOM. While allowing 41,077 others to travel.

Do the morale thing and please do not vote for these MHK's.

Some of my Correspondence to IOM Government

In the next few pages are some of the correspondence between the Isle of Man and Myself. At times my anger towards an uncaring Manx Government will be pretty obvious and my choice of words, well let's say not my best, but you can be your own judge and jury on that.

When your back is up against the wall and you're pushed into a corner by an uncaring Manx Government it is easy to lose control. I would go so far as to say this situation has drastically affected my mental health.

I know many families who are in the same situation as me, their mental health has been drastically affected. And as you will see in a communication from the Health Minister, he really does not give a toss about people, which is extremely sad. If Government health official does not care, who will? And the classic email from the Manx General Attorney, demonstrates how these people in a position of power believe that they are better than the commoner.

I have been informed of people who have moved to the Isle of Man in pretence of moving or working there so that they can visit their families. But immediate family should not have to do this. Immediate family have a humanistic right to visit their families on the Isle of Man. And no Government in the world should have any right whatsoever to stop immediate family getting access for nearly nine months and counting.

There is not a minute that goes past that I don't think of doing something similar to what our hero Dale and his Jet Ski have done. But it should not have to come to this. Moreover, the Manx Government and each individual MHK that supported this stance will be held responsible and accountable.

But I believe my fight to get access to the Isle of Man to visit my sons and grandchildren is the righteous one. I do take Covid seriously and there is no way I would ever put my family or any others at risk either off or on the Isle of Man from Covid.

I'm not proud of calling anyone a scumbag, but in reality there are times when a person or persons do fall under that title and as such they need to be called for what they really are. This might appear offensive to them, but in reality if they fit the definition then they surely do fit the name, offensive or not.

I believe in true equality, true justice and I believe that regardless of your skin colour, sexuality, creed, religion or believes, you are entitled to equality and a fundamental freedom of justice and freedom from harm. The vulnerable of this world are sadly forgotten and the people who create this vulnerability or allow this vulnerability to continue are also scumbags. The Black Life's Matter movement has highlighted around the world that vulnerable groups are the ones paying the ultimate penalty. We cannot let a Manx Government away with their mental health abuses.

On Thursday, December 10, 2020, 08:03:39 PM GMT, Ashford, David (MHK) wrote:

Dear Dave,

Thank you very much for your email. Taking each of your points in turn:

1) Yes, I do believe the island has taken the right approach in relation to borders. It is regrettable that such measures have had to be taken but we are in uncharted territory with the pandemic the like of which has not been seen since 1919. Our primary responsibility as elected members is to protect the health and well-being of the island and its residents. I firmly believe the actions taken have done so. As a nation we have no social distancing, we have achieved a Covid free community, most of our economy can operate as normal and people have been able to go about their daily lives as they did prior to the

pandemic. The island is in a unique position compared to most countries in the world and the reinstatement of widespread community transmission would be a disaster for the island from both a health, economic and wellbeing point of view.

As with other countries around the world residents have a right to enter the country to which they live, there is no such automatic right for people who do not reside in a particular country. The island is also not alone in its approach, other countries also limit due to the pandemic entry to residents only. Several others also have a ban on British nationals entering due to the U.K.s current infection rate. In fact as confirmed today, when the U.K. leaves the EU on 31st December there will be restrictions on British nationals being able to enter EU countries based on the U.K. infection rate as they will no longer be an EU member state and have automatic free movement.

The decision on entry to the island is based on risk. While a returning resident entering the island carries risk, that risk is limited as there is a natural limit on the number of people that are travelling by the population of the island. The more people you have travelling the higher the risk of contraction at ports, travel from and to ports from isolation, an accidental breach of isolation etc. All of our decisions are based around the U.K. infection rate which hopefully will decline further which will then allow us to move to 3A of our border policy which will allow family to visit.

2) Who enters the U.K. and on what terms is a matter for the U.K. Government, who decide their own border policy. Because the island is Covid free in the community the U.K. Government has taken the decision that Manx residents can enter the U.K. without isolation requirements, which is a decision for them.

In conclusion I would just like to say that it is fully recognised that this is a difficult time for many people being separated from their loved ones. I had personally hopes we would have been in a position to move to 3A before Christmas but with the current infection rate in the UK being where it currently is the risk is too high and would almost certainly lead to infections on the island even if 14 day isolation is observed. The situation will be reviewed early in the New Year and hope at that time the infection rate has declined enough as I would like nothing more than to be able to announce that people can safely bring their loved ones into the island.

Hon. David Ashford MHK, Minister for Health & Social Care

11TH December 2020, my reply to David's Ashcroft's

Dear Mr Ashcroft, (MHK of Health)

Definition of a Scumbag as per Collins dictionary: a very unpleasant person who has done something **dishonest** or **unacceptable.**

The fact that you have allowed almost 50% of your population to travel since 1st April 2020 in a global pandemic without allowing immediate family member's access to IOM for over ten months is disgusting, **unacceptable** and immoral. The fact that you tried to use the no travel as a main criteria to stop immediate family access is dishonest. The fact that you have broken international human rights, humanity and provided no justice as outlined in a previous email to Manx Government is **Dishonest** and **Unacceptable.** As such my use of the word Scumbag is acceptable and justifiable.

Mr Ashford, Firstly I would like to thank you for your extremely quick response to my email and thank you to Minister Cregeen who confirmed that David's response was "succinct" and that he supports Mr Ashcroft, it's a pity that he could not find the time to make a more fulfilling reply rather than fogging it off to his secretary to do for him.

I remember the days when a person moving to the Isle of Man was treated unfairly and was abused on regular bases by some residents and Government ministers with xenophobic remarks such as "you are only a come over, etc." Well you know all about that, do you remember that? But it's in the past, true?

No, the same is being done via our global Covid Pandemic. Your Government has become bigoted and self-centered and is basically saying screw everyone else in the UK and the world while you bask in your glory and the misery of all other nations.

You do realise that it has been ten months and counting since you have allowed immediate family access to the IOM, right? Mr Ashford you're supposed to be the Manx Mental Health Guru yet my degree in psychology and within the realm of adverse childhood experiences highlights all too well that what you are doing is detrimental to the mental health of the people being affected by your unrealistic and draconian measures.

You are sadly mistaken and incorrect in your statement that the rest of the world are doing the same as you. You are fooling yourself, your Government and your residents, there are no other countries in the world that has stopped immediate family access for over ten months, **NOT ONE COUNTRY. Ops I lied, yes there is, it's called the Isle of Man.**

Within the ongoing global pandemic you would think that countries would stick together, however the Manx Government have displayed selfishness beyond believe and its uncompressible how your Government thinks its entitled to do so. The fact that you are an offshore tax haven does not give you the right to neglect your international duties of human rights, and justice, to which I have been denied as outlined in another email to your Chief Minister.

Your comments of look at how good the IOM is doing compared to its UK is a kick in the guts, especially when the UK are allowing you to travel back and forth. Really who do you think you are? And you have the audacity to rub it in by saying it's party time in the IOM as per pre Covid days, while the rest of the world suffer and continue its attempts to achieve at least some sort of normality is disgusting, hypocritical and your Government is displaying a total lack of humanity or concern in a time of a global pandemic for others. All done while you still misuse the goodwill of the UK, the UK allows your residents to leave and come back. You have sent a clear message to the world that the Isle of Man is rich and affluent and fuck everyone else.

Your patting yourself on the back is degrading, disgusting and a few other swear slang words that you are not worthy of saying, while you watch the UK and other countries suffer. Your Government are the scum of this earth.

Your further dig at the UK on Brexit is another hypocritical and derogative remark while you still continue to let 50% of your population travel to and from the UK while allowing not one UK national entry. Disgusting and immoral. And to set the matter right, the UK's European partners have never once nor will they stop any UK national from going to their country for over ten months, like the Isle of Man did to the UK. Your Government's tactic against anyone entering the Isle of Man, especially immediate family gives the Manx Government the "Scumbag" title.

Fathers and mothers have rights and they should have at a bare minimum the exact same rights that some person wanting to move to the island for work or to start a new home for the first time, or a returning resident.

Every time a resident leaves and returns it is a risk. Do you know that the number of fathers and mothers wanting to come to the IOM is far, far less than the number of people currently travelling to the IOM on a monthly bases? Therefore, immediate family visiting the island with strict self-isolation is a lot less risky than that of returning residents, new workers and new residents wanting to live on the island. As such your logic to not allow immediate family is non-existent and is a total fabricated excuse to make it sound as if your remarks are plausible to appease an audience that is gullible.

The IOM has a population of 83,314 (IOM Government Numbers, 2020)

Number of passengers travelled to and from IOM for 1st April 2020 to 30th November 2020 = 41,077

That equates to 49% of the population on the Isle of Man has travelled in a global pandemic.

No other country including the UK has had that number of its population travel while in this global Covid pandemic. The Manx Government have proven without a shadow of a doubt that you care nothing for your neighbours. You are hiding under that umbrella because your Covid numbers are that low and you believe you are superior to all others.

You can't even let a miniscule number of immediate family onto the island while you allow almost ½ of your population to take advantage of the UK generosity and travel in a global pandemic. That's what you call a scumbag tactic.

Dave Smith

Tuesday 15ᵗʰ December: Sent to newspapers and Manx Government

Please help me in my plight to get immediate family access to the Isle of Man. The news report today of the Scottish Jet ski man attempting to visit IOM highlights the mental abuse that the Manx Government are doing to immediate family on and off the Island. I have been denied access to see my sons and grandchildren, all while the Manx Government continue to allow over 49% of its population to enter and leave the Isle of Man. Immediate family pose less of a risk than returning residents. I have been denied legal counsel with breaks international rules on justice. The Manx Government are breaking European and international human rights.

No reply received to above letter

15th December 2020: Sent to Chief Minister

In the light of the ridiculous court case and conviction against a person obviously suffering from a mental health issue with regards to your draconian and double standard Covid regulations is nonsense. His drastic action to seek what every person in this world has a right to, could have resulted in that person's death. I'm talking about Jet Ski man from Scotland.

This is further proof of the mental health strain that you are putting on people that are desperate to see family. All done while you continue to abuse the UK's goodwill of letting over 41,077 people travel to and from the island during the period of 1st April 2020 and 30th November 2020 and yet no one immediate family members are allowed access.

I'm giving the Manx Government notice that it and each member of your Government will be held liable and accountable for any person who suffers an injury or dies from their attempts to get to the Isle of Man shores to visit loved ones.

It is obvious that your draconian measures are hampering the mental health of many and this will not be tolerated.

Dave Smith

No reply received from Chief Minister, but a reply from Walter H Wannenburg on 16th December 2020 was received.

Dear Mr Smith

I refer to your recent series of correspondence addressed to, inter alia, the Chief Minister and his private secretary and comprising:

Your letter of 3 July 2020 addressed to "Members of the Manx Government"

Your subsequent emails 5 July 2020 (timed at 17:49), 1 October 2020 (10:06), 5 October 2020 (13:56), 6 October 2020 (15:34), 12 October 2020 (10:19), 24 November 2020 (14:55), 26 November 2020 (21:10), 30 November 2020 (14:00), 9 December 2020 (13:55), 10 December 2020 (11:41), 10 December 2020 (16:37), 11 December 2020 19:52 and 15 December 2020 (20:26).

Your second email of 10 December 2020 (addressed to all Ministers / Government departments and media outlets) received a reasoned and substantive response from Minister Ashford: your reply made plain that you disagreed with his comments as is your right. Unhappily however your correspondence AS SCHEDULED ABOVE has routinely gone beyond simple disagreement and has been intemperate and on occasion abusive.

While it is understood that the present travel restrictions result in difficulties for you (and very many other people), they are nonetheless approved by Tynwald which has regarded same as a necessary and proportionate response to the pandemic. The full restrictions can be accessed at

https://legislation.gov.im/cms/images/LEGISLATION/SUBORDINATE/2020/2020/0279/EmergencyPowersCoronavirusEntryRestrictionsNo.2Regulations2020_6.pdf and

https://legislation.gov.im/cms/images/LEGISLATION/SUBORDINATE/2020/2020-0370/EmergencyPowersCoronavirusContinuationNo.2Regulations2020_8.pdf.

The measures implemented (regarded as striking an appropriate balance between human rights and emergency response requirements) do not depend in any way upon the legislative steps taken in any other jurisdiction whether in the United Kingdom or the Channel Islands (or elsewhere) and so your comments as to reciprocity between the Island and those countries are not relevant. For the record, your various allegations that the travel restriction provisions constitute, inter alia, "double standards and corruption", "violation of human rights" and "tyranny of the highest degree…" are denied.

Additionally I have noted your several references to the likelihood of you pursuing legal proceedings against the Isle of Man Government (and "against each member of Government on an individual basis") and that you will be claiming sums of, variously £10million (12.10.20), £1million (09.12.20), £25million (10.12.20).

In the circumstances I have advised that there is no benefit in continuing to respond to your correspondence, and you should not expect any further replies. Should you decide to instruct legal representatives and / or issue formal legal proceedings, they may be served at the Attorney General's Chambers at the address below marked for my attention.

Yours

Walter Wannenburgh, H.M. Solicitor General, Isle of Man

My Reply to Walter Wannenburgh, cc to Chief Minister, 16th Dec 2020.

I agree, I see no point in repeating myself either.

But regardless I will expect a reply when I correspond. And I still hold the Isle of Man in contempt of international human rights and of International Justice to which there is no time expiration on my claim for compensation. Moreover, I will be looking for compensation for every immediate family member that has been affect by your double standards and abuse to immediate family.

The fact that you are allowing any tom (actual residents), dick (new and possible residents) and harry (people with the money wanting to buy a house to further your rich and affluent society) to arrive on the IOM while not allowing a few immediate family members is your outright acceptance of guilt and acceptance of my compensation claims.

It is extremely sad, that even up to now, your Government cannot make any exceptions and allow a small number of immediate family members access. After all you have allowed 41,077 Manx people to travel back and forth since April 2020 to November 2020 and you have the audacity to tell me I'm wrong. 49% of your population have travelled during Covid. Get real!

Dave

Dear Mr Wannenburgh, Sent 21st December 2020

Further to your email, and your pointing out various claim amounts. I just want to clarify that my claim against the Isle of Man Government now stands at twenty five million pounds sterling, plus the same amount for each person who has been affected by your fraudulent and basic breach of human rights.

Hope that makes it crystal clear for you.

Dave Smith

Ok, so Walters reply above was the usual legal nonsense reply: But here is the main point. I contacted every law firm on the Isle of Man as per the Manx Law Society. **Not one legal firm** could represent me on my quest to take litigation against the Manx Government.

As a result I have been denied justice as defined by the United Nations and International rights of an individual to be provided with legal counsel in that country.

So not only have they broken International Human rights but they have not allowed justice to ensue. Hence, why Jet Ski man Dale has had to take drastic steps towards achieving his own method of justice. When a Government takes away your justice, then justice does not exist and as such each individual affected, is entitled to take Justice into their own hands. That is a fundamental right of being a human on earth, though Governments and their legal systems will deny you this right.

Conclusion and my Correspondence in a nutshell:

Yes, I'm sorry being forced to reduce myself to the level that the Manx Government have displayed in its stance against immediate families. Yes, I'm sorry that I felt the desperate need to call someone a scumbag. What I have said and what Dale did on his Jet Ski is from a mental health desperation of wanting the natural right to visit loved ones on the Isle of Man.

Desperation makes a person do things that they don't want to do but are now forced to do. The Manx Government have put immediate family under attack and when a person or persons do that then you retaliate in a way to try and facilitate change. However, by doing so each side of this fence become resolved not to let the other win. You can see this mentality occurring throughout the world and with major world leaders. Guess who are let down with this type of thinking? Yep, it's the vulnerable. The vulnerable suffer at the hands of people and Governments who do not do the appropriate and morally right thing, regardless of consequences to themselves.

How many times have you read stories about the person who puts their life at risk to safe another? Well not the Manx Government, you aren't getting on their lifeboat.

However, when you are fighting for your rights against a Government that pertains to be your overarching authority then that fight becomes quite unique, and you are brainwashed into believing that what they do is for your best. When deep down you know that this is just not right, nor is it ethical. The Manx Government have 100% proved that what they are doing towards immediate family and still allowing 41,077 of their residents to travel, displays a total lack of any ethics whatsoever and is harming a vulnerable portion of society.

I have clearly demonstrated other ways that immediate family could be given entry to the Isle of Man while ensuring the safety of Manx residents. I have also pointed out that no other country in the world has taken such a draconian attitude and banned all of their resident's immediate family for nine months and counting.

It is therefore without a shadow of a doubt that the Isle of Man Government have inflicted grave mental health issues on their resident's immediate families and as such must be held accountable for these discriminations and international violations within the International arena of justice.

It is obvious that the Manx Government have attempted to brain wash their residents with the fear of keeping non Manx off the island so that they cannot catch Covid from them. This is not only narrow minded but stinks of double standards when they allow 49% of their population to travel to and from the UK under Covid. Do the Manx Government honestly believe that immediate family members wanting to arrive on the Island have super-duper Covid infecting genes that returning self-isolating residents don't have?

When you consider this fact there is no difference whatsoever between a self-isolating resident and a self-isolating immediate family member on the Isle of Man. As such the Manx Government have done a fantastic job at brain washing the public.

I would like to end this section with the advice of don't take peoples word, research information for yourself, become empowered and look for the truth and equality in all that you do and above all fight for freedom, human rights, and fight for the vulnerable people in our world.

To Dale, you are my hero, you are the hero of many on the Isle of Man and indeed throughout the world. History will record what you did as a fight for justice and to be close to the people you love. No Government have any legal right to stop immediate family visiting, regardless of their man made legislation. Birth rights supersede any manufactured legal crap.

To the Manx Government, shame on you, you have let the Manx people down, you have let the International community that support you down. You are an utter disgrace and the Manx people need to use their vote. Do not re-elect these people.

On your death and onward universal passage there are no confessions acceptable, you will be judged purely by your acts of humanity, by the correcting of injustice and inequality and by the way you have treated the vulnerable of this world. And with that statement in mind I know exactly where the Manx Cabinet ministers are going.

While you may be able to sleep at night comfortable in your beds, your day of judgement will come faster than what you think. Look at your life, what age are you now in this moment in time? Whatever age you are now, that time has passed in a flick of your fingers, and with the next flick of your fingers you will face judgement and your judgement will not be based on your so called motive of keeping the few safe but on the others that you allowed to sink on your global pandemic ship.

Robert C from twitter asked me why my children could not leave the Island and visit me. Firstly, that would not be fair, why should they have to leave, just to appease a Manx Government? Secondly, my sons work and can't get the needed four weeks off from their work to do this. My grandchildren are at school on the IOM. Therefore, in a nutshell that option is not feasible at all. Whereas I can go to the IOM.

Scan the QR image below to visit the Manx Government Covid Information website.

Update to Exiting a Pandemic:

A report from National Geographic, December 2020 stated, *"It's apparently humankind's fate never to stop writing the history of pandemics. No matter how often they occur – and they do occur with great frequency – we collectively refuse to think about them until circumstances demand it."*

	At 17th December 2020	At 20th May 2020
Global Cases of Covid:	75,204,485	5,018,657
Total of deaths:	1,666,636	325,673
% who died from Covid, based on total number of cases:	2.2%	6.5%

From the statistics above you can see that in a space of seven months the dramatic increase of the number of cases and deaths. However the death % has dropped quite considerably. Is that due to false reporting or is it the effect of being able to isolate those most vulnerable to the virus and give them more protection?

Nine months on and many countries of the world are still batting to keep Covid under control. There have been several lockdowns and then "circuit breakers" and Tiers 1, 2 and 3 and so forth. One day your business is open and the next day it is closed. Stay at home, don't stay at home, don't go to work, go to work, and don't go to work but send your children to school and so forth… The leaders haven't set out any clear pathway on what should be done. And Governments are finding it hard to keep infection rates down.

As such Governments have been totally irresponsible and are accountable for the deaths that have occurred due to their mishandling of a global pandemic. If the leaders of the world had actually cared about the wellbeing of people and had put them first over that of a materialistic economy, then they would have locked down at the same time as China for four weeks. And the result of that would have made a drastic difference to the number of deaths and the world's economies would more secure than what they are now. But alas, as we all know sadly that did not happen. Now we are in and out of lockdowns with no real clarity of Covid free in sight. But there is now a December 2020 vaccine developed from different pharmaceuticals. I do hope that these companies are not profiteering off the back of people's misery, if so it must be halted.

People need to wear masks, people need to maintain a social distance, if we all do those simple of tasks it does not remove your freedom but it protects yourself and others. Please care for others and do these simple requests.

During some of the lockdowns schools remained open. This has mixed views depending on your outlook and experience. If I put on my psychology and adverse childhood experience hat then I would have to agree that school children in some instances should be at school. However, the current way schools are currently operating is detrimental to the health of the children at school, and the virus will spread quicker between school, family, friends and co-workers. If a school child has Covid unknown and infects the father or mother who then goes to work and spreads it to another. You get the drift. No lockdown as is being currently carried out will stop this form reoccurring if children are forced to go to school.

Government states: "School children will go to school during the current lockdowns." Announcement: "With School children not being at school over Christmas, it is likely the "R" rate will go down." Do they not realise what has been said? They have just confirmed that forcing children to go to school will imply huge increases in infection spread. So why do it? This is additional proof that the powers to be really do not have a clue and are avoiding common sense and other scientific advice that could make a difference if applied.

The health authorities have outlined that children might not display the systems but will be carriers. And when there are thirty to a class, safe distancing does not exist. Even when school finish for the day you see hundreds pouring out in an extreme close proximity. The risk of infection in these circumstance is a vicious circle, it will go around and around.

Are the UK Government trying to silently introduce herd mentality via the schools and have now been caught out?

The solution to children going to school is: To drastically reduce the numbers in a class by over ½. One half attends school in the morning and the other half in the afternoon. Remote learning is done when each half is at home. Yep, this implies ensuring that all children in all groups in society have access to the internet and a computer. And that's not much to ask for either is it?

Several vaccines are being released with no real scientific knowledge of what the future will hold regardless of being vaccinated or not, and they have done limited vaccine testing. Cancer drugs have been kept on the shelf for years, yet Covid vaccines are out already and it hasn't even been a year?

Business that have been around for decades such as Debenhams and others are going out of business. Where is the help from the Government for these businesses? The Government have made idiotic rules and have demonstrated that they certainly are not qualified to handle this pandemic. If they had of followed China's lead in January 2020 and the world locked down their country totally, as like China, then we would not be in this position today, nor would the world have had as many deaths.

It is quite possible that living with Covid will become the new norm. As such we must protect those that are in the vulnerable and essential worker groups. We must research and find an effective vaccine that can easily be mutated to rid humanity of any new strains. But we should not forget about our other international duties such as protecting the vulnerable of the world.

We also need to halt climate change otherwise the next pandemic will make Covid look like a kindergarten party. Halting climate change will incur a high cost, we cannot continue to live our lives as we do at present. With a growing population soon to reach 8 billion people, will put the world's natural resources at breaking point. We cannot burn fossil fuel any longer. Each person on earth must stand up and become a climate activist. Politian's and Governments must come under immense pressure to change their ways. Use your vote, make your vote count, and get rid of Politian's that don't put our climate first.

But it is not all doom and gloom, many companies that were once polluters are changing to become green and sustainable companies. Renewable energies are now cheaper and are becoming more available than fossil fuel energy. People are starting to eat healthier and reduce their meat intake. Our throw away culture needs to be remodelled towards becoming a reuse and recycle community.

Don't buy water in plastic throwaway bottles. Plastic was once the making of our industrious future, but that future has now caught up with us. Oceans and its inhabitants including our land animal stock have ingested plastic particles. Plastics have now entered the human food chain.

Cars can now be powered with green electric. Airbus and others are developing green and sustainable aircraft. The future can be bright, but every person must keep up the pressure to do more today, because tomorrow will be too late for your children's future.

Governments need to offer massive discounts so that the ordinary person in the street can afford an electric vehicle, or a solar panels to power their home and so forth. It cannot just be for the rich. This assistance and discount could form part of a means testing, so if you have the money you will pay full price. If you are an ordinary "joe" then you should get massive discount in the way of free grants and other types of support.

We must help the vulnerable throughout the world, because they are the ones that will suffer the most in a climate emergency. The vulnerable around the world are the ones that has suffered more during Covid. The vulnerable are the ones that are in a position of being depraved from freedom and equality. Please fight for justice. On your death bed you will be only judged on your humanity to others and not your wealth.

New Virus Strain (Publicly announced by UK PM Boris Johnson)

Boris created a new Tier, called Tier 4, just to address the increases in the new strain of the virus. Johnson announced that this new strain can have faster and easier transmission rates, but will not affect you in any different way as is present. I mentioned in my book in May 2020 that not enough is known about Covid and that there is a high chance of it mutating.

The UK Government stated that the current Covid vaccines will still be effective against this new strain. However, some countries are jumping on the "I'm so scared" band wagon to halt travel in the endeavour to stop the strain from getting to their country. Some Questions that need answered:

1) Why is the UK the only country currently with this new strain? Could it be that the UK are the cleanest nation and with all their sanitising etc., that Covid has become partially immune to this over indulgence in Covid warfare? After all medical staff are always making it crystal clear, don't overdo antibiotics, if you do the "virus DNA" changes to counter act what humans are doing to stop it in the first place.

2) Countries refused to lockdown at the critical time, as what China did. Other countries did not do this because it meant their economies would suffer. Now look how shoddier the world's economies are now. It's crazy, and a massive mismanagement of a pandemic by world Government leaders.

3) So, if Covid managed to mutate to a new strain in the London area, why did this occur? And why specifically London or the UK? Find the reason and you help the world.

4) So, if London or the UK managed to witness the development of a new strain, why do other world Government leaders not understand that their countries virus strain could mutate to become their local version? Any new strain could be based on their demographics and the law of biochemistry and change patterns.

5) The UK Government knew about this new strain long before they put London into tier 3 (December 2020,) then a week later they announced a new tier 4, which London was immediately put into. Was this a ploy of the UK Government to mitigate London protesters, as most Londoners believed that from the 30th December they would go back to tier 2? Or was it to offset any possible retaliation by the UK's departing BREXIT neighbours. Even the idiotic North of Ireland are trying to jump on the panic bandwagon and practise "ostracism" in their attempt to stop other members of the UK from travelling to Northern Ireland. Pity they too did not lock down when China announced their lockdown. Again, shabby devolved leadership and this latest move is primarily designed as a political move rather than a move for the true interests of people. And remember this is coming from the mouths of leaders who want schools still to return while everyone else isolates. Hypercritical and utter nonsense, they really have no clue on how to operate or deal with a Pandemic effetely.

6) Time Spector, professor of genetic epidemiology (11/12/2020) Speaking at a Royal Society of Medicine event argued, *"This on-off business is a total disaster, and we should avoid it…It would be a big mistake if London goes into tier 3…We need to think about these tier systems. The whole point should be the capacity of the*

NHS to deal with it locally. At the moment, according to our data, London has plenty of spare capacity [in hospitals]. We know we aren't going to get rid of this virus before the vaccine, so we need to make sure the NHS is under control and that people over the age of 60 are not getting it at bad rates and have some clear criteria...the Government should stop treating people like "cattle" to be led and instead give them better information and trust them to do the right thing. "Just having this league table of who is being relegated and promoted and this on-off effect is madness," he added. "We need a much more consistent pattern that we can all relate to...tell people the truth and what is going on in your area" BMJ 2020;371:m4798

Moreover, **questions need answered** and if the virus can mutate in the UK then it will do so in every other city around the world, regardless of what you do to stop the transmission. The main reason for short-term lockdowns is to ease the pressure on health care authorities, as they cannot help everyone if they are subjected to more admissions than they can realistically handle.

However, the most effective way is to isolate the vulnerable and those most susceptible to sever infection and death from this virus. It has been proven throughout the world and even in the USA, the people who live in poverty or are vulnerable, or have a lack of access to health foods and sanitation are the ones who become the groups with the highest infection and death rates.

Do world leaders need a neon sign stretching across the skies of our earth saying? "Help those in poverty and whom are vulnerable," before they realise that the rich again are the ones who can ride out this Covid pandemic and get the better health care? In the USA Trumps top aids and non Covid believers are the ones getting the Covid Vaccine first. What type of people are they, really? The vaccine should be given to every vulnerable group and **ALL** essential services worker first. Shop assistants risk their life's on a daily bases with the huge number of people whom they deal with. Childminders, school teachers and nursery staff are essential. Doctors and nurses are essential. Any person who performs an essential service dealing with members of the public should be recognised as an essential worker and as such should be one of the first to receive the vaccine.

Another major question that needs answered: **When a person is vaccinated, do they stop becoming carriers of the Covid virus? Do they stop transmitting the Covid virus once vaccinated?**

The CDC (2020) has stated, *"There is no evidence that getting a flu vaccination increases your risk of getting sick from coronavirus, like the one that causes COVID-19."* They further said, *"…flu vaccination will vary, depending on factors like the characteristics of the person being vaccinated (for example, their health and age), what influenza viruses are circulating that season and, potentially, which type of flu vaccine was used."* Which instigates a further questions.

- Will the Covid vaccine become the same type of vaccinated solution as the current flu vaccinations?

- Will the Covid vaccine be required on a regular bases? And if yes what are the side-affects or consequences of people taking so many different vaccinations?

The CDC also reported that, *"many people at higher risk from flu also seem to be at higher risk from COVID-19."*

In a nutshell, will Covid vaccinated people no longer be carriers and become transmitter free? If not then they too must continue to wear a mask and practice social distancing. This statement from the CDC about infecting others after receiving the flu vaccine is not exactly clear on that matter, *"Getting vaccinated yourself **may also** protect people around you, including those who are more vulnerable to serious flu illness."* Source of above: https://www.cdc.gov/flu/prevent/misconceptions.htm

Covid Panic and Cancer

While the world panics about Covid, **let's spare a thought for the estimated 9.5 million people that will die each year from cancer worldwide. That's around 26,000 people each day and represents 1 out of every 6 other types of deaths.** Yet cancer treatment and hospitalisation has been neglected in the era of the World's Leaders negligent handling of the Covid Pandemic.

The burning and use of fossil fuels has been attributed to pollution and air quality which has resulted in millions being inflicted by many forms of cancer. Yet the world does not panic, you continue to go about your daily duties polluting the earth will CO_2. But along comes Covid with a higher survival rate than cancer and leaders panic the world, while carrying out pathetic measures, which most are too late.

The only way forward is to scrap our current economic model and say good bye and good riddance to the mega wealthy and introduce a humanistic circular economy. An economy based on greenness and sustainability that does not endanger our planet and the world's biodiversity. By putting people and our planets Health before wealth is your only hope for salvation on your death bed. Your children's future depends on how quick we act today.

Acting tomorrow is a pure excuse and if COP26 does not produce immediate and drastic actions then the world will witness a mass protest.

Stopping pollution and unhealthy eating will cut down cancer cases dramatically. Likewise a healthier planet = a healthier person = a better immune system to beat Covid.

Covid is not the problem, people are the problem. You have been led to a materialistic gate that you now believe you can do anything that you want. Humans are not superior, so stop being assholes and start doing things that will actually benefit your neighbours and the vulnerable around the world. Borders create injustices and wealth creates global misery and while the rich get richer the masses get poorer. The current economic model is now defunct to save earth and if it continues then the people in poverty and those vulnerable groups will be the ones that face the most deaths and injustices. And when that happens humans have just become in-humane.

The only true way forward is towards creating a "sustainable and humanistic circular economy." And to do this will be an uphill battle against a minority of people and it will be that same minority that holds the wealth and hence the unfair laws that you will be scrutinised under.

Offshore tax havens are one classic example, the majority of Manx residents can't even afford a house of their own as the rich and affluent have forced house prices through the roof. The rich and affluent get a better class of the same law that we all are supposed to have.

EXITING A PANDEMIC

RESEARCH ON A VIRUS, CLIMATE CHANGE AND EXIT

DAVE SMITH

Exiting a Lockdown

Research on a Virus, Climate Change and Exit

First Published, May 2020

The USA are threatening to stop funding going to the World Health Organisation.

On 15th April, 2020 President Trump delayed funding to the World Health Organisation, what an IDIOT-1 he is. In a time of need throughout the world Trump has acted in a childish manner while in reality it was Trump and his administration that botched up the USA's own lock-down measures. The USA Government are ultimately responsible for the death of 86,937 (as at 15th May 2020). Plus the USA's lack of immediate action has led to many other deaths in other countries as they still allowed people to travel to other countries. The USA and other countries could have locked down at the same time as China and not up to 3 months later. So, don't be too quick to blame others for your countries lack of action.

Scan the image below to get a look at the virus timeline of events. Understanding a timeline could help assist with any decision and actions for an exit from a pandemic. It can also clarify some issues of concern. The purpose of this book is to provide you with information and resources where you can get verification and make your own informed research from reliable sources. Hopefully this book will act as a seed for your thoughts to grow into a realisation that if we do not act now to halt climate change, then this current pandemic will only serve as a window into an unrecognisable world that you have allowed your children to inherit.

https://www.thinkglobalhealth.org/article/updated-timeline-coronavirus

Scan the QR codes below to see what the UK, USA and others lockdown phased exit roadmaps are. I will update the image content as they become available.

They will also include any relevant changes that the countries make to their published exit roadmaps.

UK	USA

Other Countries	Ireland

UK Government advice changed from Herd Immunity to:

Stay at Home…Save Life's…Anyone can Spread Coronavirus

USA Governments Initially advice by Trump:
We have it totally under control…It may get smaller or bigger, but let's see first (Their initial inaction cost 86,000 human lives so far)

Then Trump ill advises: On Hydroxychloroquine as a treatment and next was to inject yourself with chemicals (To both: DO NOT DO THIS - Amazingly despite all of his blunders and ill advice from his advisors Trump and his administration are still in power) Trump has been trying to rally himself as the heroic leader of the global pandemic, possibly for the next presidential election. But in reality he failed miserably. Perhaps if the virus had dollars protruding, he would have done a better job?

Pollution, COVID-19 and Saving Lives

On March 16th 2020, it was announced that research has demonstrated the impact of CO_2 pollution and its effects on the Chinese population. In this report they estimate it that 77,000 lives have been saved because of the China Lock-down (in China alone.) Therefore the lives saved in china is 16.6 times more than the COVID-19 deaths.

What does that above statement say to any ordinary individual, never mind our Government and leaders? I really do not think you need to have any university degree or any intelligence. In fact I would guarantee that even plankton could come to the same conclusion. That conclusion is, if we halt pollution we will save millions of lives around the world.

As at May 15th, 2020, the global deaths from coronavirus were 303,996. Therefore, if we take the above analogy for all countries throughout the world, and if they were to lock-down with the same furiousness as China, then the world could have saved almost 5 million unnecessary deaths because of drastic reductions in world pollution.

Therefore, we have to question Governments, leaders, Politian's and political scientific advisors with two principal questions and probably many other sub-questions.

- **Question 1**: Why is there no lock-down or drastic steps being taken to halt co2, and other pollutions. The current climate change reductions by countries around the world is painfully slow, so slow that they are putting your children and their children's lives at extreme risk.

- **Question 2**: Is the slowness of attending to climate change because of a desired reduction in the world's population?

- **Likely answer:** wealth and economy is being put before that of Health and Human Prosperity.

Sadly, countries' economies will shape and form the roadmap and strategic action plan for any exit from the current pandemic lock-down.

In order to understand and formulate any attempt

At an exit or roadmap for exiting a 'pandemic lockdown,' we must first consider all the facts. How the virus was created, how we can stop these types of viruses from starting again, and how we can develop vaccinations quicker for the future. This will be an ongoing task for the world's medical and scientific teams.

The world has been given an ideal opportunity to build a defence and strategy for developing a plan of action to halt viruses in their spreading tracks. Despite many leaders and Politian's in the past saying an epidemic is on the horizon, countries have disregarded this and spent more money on warfare as heard throughout the world by president Trumps May 2020 statement saying that "America has a super-duper space weapon." This pandemic and lockdown will surly serve as a sign to Governments that we need to transcend from a wealth economy to a Health economy. This book will start with investigating coronavirus, climate change and an exit from lockdown.

Lockdown's have not been fully road mapped, yet the post-mortem of the pandemic events have now begun. The UK Government are being blamed for putting the NHS first before that of the care homes, which house most of the vulnerable. Close to my heart are the shop workers who were left to attend to thousands of people on a daily basis without any of the PPE that the NHS had.

It would appear that the UK Government worked on the sentiments of the people and used the NHS as yet another pandemic BREXIT showcase, while leaving most people who needed their help both on PPE equipment but also legislation to protect such Individuals. While we are all eternally grateful for the work that the NHS do, we also need to reflect on what other front-line workers have had to endure without the necessary PPE equipment and resources.

The other major post-mortem that can and will affect the world, are the statements made by President Trump on his personal use and his indirect recommendation that every person should use the anti-malaria drug hydroxychloroquine to combat COVID-19. Despite medical advice, he said it was harmless. Trump has proven repeatedly that he is a danger to the world.

Trumps other inflammatory statements include renaming the virus and that punishments should be handed out to those responsible for this virus are not only outrageous, it is a roadmap to war and confrontation.

The president of America has been termed a pathological liar by many that work and know him. He is a president that has never accepted any blame whatsoever, and passing the blame on to others is like water off a ducks back for Donald. Trump and his family are still under criminal investigation and history will show that Trump and his administration were directly responsible for allowing the virus to claim so many lives in America.

What you will need to use this book

This is an interactive book with many additional links to videos, research and information. It also includes a few pages of activities to keep everyone at home busy while you endure your lock-down.

You will require:

- An Internet connection. (To scan QR images or click on hyperlinks to view videos and other research.)

- A QR reader so you can scan the images. [If you see any advertisements, then they are part of the QR reader that you downloaded and not my QR images, mine are 100% add free.]

COVID-19 LIVE UPDATES

Scan QR image below to view a LIVE UPDATE with full statistics for all countries.

https://qrs.ly/z5bddgo

Rolling Update on COVID-19 from WHO

Scan QR code below to be kept up to date with latest COVID-19 Information from the World Health Organisation. (WHO)

https://qrs.ly/z3bcxyd

Scan the QR image below to get a complete update of COVID-19 including advice and links from the NHS and other websites.

This website presents the information in a good format while utilising information from reliable, health and Government websites.

https://qrs.ly/babduah

UK Government Latest Updates on information for the public

https://qrs.ly/dqbe4rk

European Centre for Disease Prevention and Control,

https://qrs.ly/15be4rl

GOV Ireland: Latest updates on COVID-19

https://qrs.ly/p8be4rp

Centre for Disease control & Prevention (CDC) Latest Updates

https://qrs.ly/hfbe4rr

wealth

Throughout this book you will listen to me rant about Health before wealth and you will notice that wealth is always spelt with a small letter "w" as it does not deserve to be capitalised. However, I would like to point out I'm not against free trade or bettering one's self per se. What I'm getting at is ending excessive wealth building, this does not serve anyone. Moreover, the wealth system psychologically makes you believe that such people deserve this wealth. In reality no one deserves such wealth. Ending billionaires and multi-millionaires needs to be a top priority. Health must come before wealth. Ending growing poverty, homelessness while increasing true equality should be a top priority. Capping the income of individuals and companies must be on the table.

The World's growing Population
Those at Risk from COVID-19

"The world's population is ageing: virtually every country in the world is experiencing growth in the number and proportion of older persons in their population."

Source https://www. https://www.un.org/en/sections/issues-depth/ageing/

World Population Prospects 2019 https://population.un.org/wpp/

COVID-19 has been described to date, as mostly affecting the elderly and vulnerable throughout the world.

As at 2019 they estimated that there were 709,000,000 people over the age of 65 in the world.

When 2050 arrives they project that there will be 1.5 billion people over the age of 65 in the world.

We must care and protect these members of our society. We need to develop a vaccine as a priority. Poverty affects everyone but more so the vulnerable groups, therefore it would be expected that more deaths could occur in areas and countries where poverty is the highest.

There are not enough statistics or results to outline how many of the elderly and vulnerable who have been infected with the virus and have died or lived. Such statistics are vital in determining how brutal the virus is towards that group of people.

It is also vital to uncover how people are catching the virus, and how is it spreading

The world's total population is 7.8 billion people, and it is growing dramatically. By 2050 they estimate that there will be 9.7 billion people sharing this planet.

It will take an alternative way of life to feed this growing population. Traditional meat farming and production is not a viable option as this is causing an even greater climate disaster.

Plant based food is one of our options, a reduction in the number of births is another.

Sadly 32 years ago Prince Philip made the following comment, *"In the event that I am reincarnated, I would like to return as a deadly virus, to contribute something to solving overpopulation."* Those words have come back to haunt him. While we can't blame him for COVID-19, we can condone his remarks as disgusting and inhumane, but such remarks are fitting of a historical monarchy or Nazis where both groups tried to do what they wanted to do.

Despite wars, famines, flu and cancer to name but a few, the world's population is still increasing dramatically.

- 40 million people died to World War 1
- 75 to 118 million people died to World War 2
- 30 to 57 million died to the Mongol conquests
- 17 to 100 million died to the 1918 flu pandemic.
- 9.6 million Worldwide deaths because of cancer each year

The above figures are staggering and sick, how can humanity allow these deaths to occur. And the above is only a small number of such deaths.

To maintain a healthy Earth and to sustain all life forms we need a radical change to human behaviour and halt climate change and injustices throughout the world.

In order for every species to live healthy on this planet we need a radical change in every aspect of human's current existence.

The changes required will be so dramatic that it will upset many people. We can no longer allow billionaires and millionaires to control our society. We can no longer allow their greed to destroy humanity and earth. We need every person to make personal sacrifices by turning away from unsustainable resources like fossil fuels etc. We need a removal of large corporations to be replaced by smaller business that will care about people and the environment.

The current model of the world's economy towards wealth does not work for the majority of the world's population. It only serves the minority of the world's population. The wealthy suck all the little people into feeding their wealth and greed. This must end to save humanity.

Malaria

The world health organisation have stated that in 2018 there were 228 million malaria cases and 405,000 deaths. On my first visit to Africa, my partner counted 200 mosquito bites on my body. I developed symptoms that included fever, headaches, chills and diarrhoea. Luckily I was treated by a local doctor and suffered no major effects. However, people who do not have enough money, which is the majority, have to take their gamble with malaria. Yet the world shuts down over coronavirus. **Help is urgently needed in African countries to stop this murderous disease.**

Facts:

- Every 2 minutes a child dies with malaria

- Unlike coronavirus, malaria's key target is those under 5 years of age. And 67% of all malaria deaths are of children under 5.

- The African region has 93% of all reported cases and 94% of the malaria deaths.

- While Donald Trump believes that a drug developed for anti-malaria is the "solution" spare a thought for all the children dying because they don't have access to hydroxychloroquine.

When I first visited Africa, the poverty overcame me, yet the Africans still kept their humanity and dignity. I was confused on how I could help when so much help was needed. So I did what Mother Teresa suggested, "If you can't feed them all, start with one." And to this day we as a family still help. You can too.

December 2020: Mutation of the Covid Virus

It has been announced that the Covid virus has mutated. Scientist have said that it is evolving but is doing so at a very slow pace as compared to the flu virus and aids. This will give more time for alternative vaccines to be produced. However, scientist have also admitted that they do not know everything at this stage and that anything is possible.

Thushan de Silva, an infectious diseases doctor at the University of Sheffield and member of the Covid-19 Genomics UK Consortium (COG-UK) said, "*This virus is evolving and that's what we expect it to do.*"

As such people still need to take the necessary precautions regardless of being one of the people who have managed to be vaccinated.

Preface

Exiting a lockdown shall look at the world's COVID-19 reduction effort as compared to the Climate emergency effort, and how we can exit from a lockdown that has affected the entire world. I have included information on Coronavirus from the World Health Organisation and other reliable sources to help you gain an insight and retrieve accurate and valuable information from the scientific health community and experts on **how to deal with COVID-19.**

The UK and Irish Governments have so far have displayed their true colours in their efforts to help their populations from financial disaster for that we applaud them. I have heard that the USA have added 2 trillion dollars for financial support. However, most of this financial aid is selected for corporations. If this is true, then Trump and his administration should be ashamed of themselves, but there again you would expect this from an administration that puts wealth before its people. But please spare a thought and give help to countries that don't have the financial ability that developed countries have. Every country is in this together, let's be united and stand together to help each other. Let's show the universe that humans can show humanity and compassion before that of wealth generation.

The universe needs to know that we can all pull together and be one. The universe needs to see an end to billionaires and excessively rich people and a switch to become a world where health, freedom and equality comes before all else. This is a defining moment for the world. Exiting a lockdown to resume what we did in the past is a demonstration to the universe that humans don't really give a fuck about earth and the people inhabited there.

We can no longer allow the wealthy to control our industries and dictate what our Governments and leaders will do. At no point in time shout billionaires be allowed to be leaders of our Governments, nor can we can allow them to fund any donations to political parties.

Since beginning to write this book, I soon discovered that it could become an endless task to complete as the mapping and dissemination of information was changing on an hourly basis. I updated COVID-19 cases and deaths on a daily basis. This also highlighted the urgent need for everyone to take this virus seriously, to practice self-isolation and only go out when necessary. While remembering to practice social distancing. **I have included QR images that will take you to websites and videos that will give you live up-to-date information.**

While we are all in the midst of this pandemic and many are suffering from anxiety and in a domain of the unknown, we cannot turn our backs on a more pressing 'future pandemic' and that's CLIMATE CHANGE. We need to embrace our current coronavirus challenges and use this knowledge to make for a better future whilst halting climate cancer.

COVID-19 is now affecting 210 countries. Staying safe should always be a top priority. COVID-19 is a new strain of the coronavirus, and scientists are still in their infancy of gathering knowledge to halt it in its future tracks. This book's contents result from research into scientific material, available data and general media and consensus.

Please know that there are many false coronavirus claims being bandied about on social media websites and fake news websites. Please be careful when reading such stories. Some are very misleading. Always do your own verification from reliable sources.

In compiling this book, I have taken research from international and local authorities. Sometimes I will make references to material from news reporting websites. I also want to state that while I talk about climate change and its effect on all of us, I'm not being light hearted about COVID-19. We should take it seriously for everyone's future wellbeing, but at the same time we have to be knowledgeable and to protect ourselves from climate change, for that will be our next pandemic.

Countries from all over the world have clarified that COVID-19 is now a pandemic. And as never witnessed before countries are going into some form of lock-down in their attempts to stop the virus until a) more is known about it and b) a vaccine can be safely made. c) Test are available and are being carried out on a massive scale. As at 24th March 2020, it was estimated that only 20% of the world is in lock-down. This is not good enough to halt the virus spreading.

I have included QR links within the book that will keep you up-to-date with all the latest COVID-19 news and developments. However, while you may feel compelled to constantly search out virus news, it is beneficial for your wellbeing if you don't do this throughout your day. Take a health break from the news and concentrate on you and your family's wellbeing, do activities and talk with each other.

A message to the people who have stockpiled: This is outrageous what you have done. What you are saying is screw everyone else as long as you are ok. This is not acceptable by any means. Supermarkets and shops should have been proactive and halted this from the very first person who went out their door with more than what they would require for 1 week and not have waited for any Government intervention. Everyone deserves the right for food, not just you.

So I would encourage all stockpiler's to either a) Donate that additional food to a food-bank or b) Share your stockpile with neighbours.

Individuals and businesses who sell products at increased prices to make a further gain or additional profits should be halted and held accountable. These people are utterly scumbags, and should be treated as such. Purchase nothing from them, name and shame them and stay away from their businesses.

Lock-downs, China locked down their country in mid-January 2020, approximately 21 days after the outbreak. Their lock-down was exactly that, it was a lock-down. *"These extreme limitations on population movement have been quite successful,"* says

In the UK, on the weekend of 21st March 2020 after the prime minister announced a semi-lock-down mostly featuring social distancing. Parks and towns were packed with people that were not practising social distancing. So the virus will continue to spread at the cost of others' lives. The PM then announced tougher measures, parks and beaches are to be closed and suggested travel for food, medicine and essential work only.

On Friday 25th March, Ireland announced a tighter control on the lock-downs, people were informed only go out for exercise or shopping and to remain within 2km of your home.

Italy was the first country to put the entire 60 million population on a total lock-down. Anyone breaking this will face up to three months in jail. Italy as at 29th March has seen 10,023 deaths.

Spain ordered a country wide lock down for a minimum of two weeks to be reassessed. You can only go out for food, medicine or essential work. Spain as at 29th March has seen 5,982 deaths.

What is further alarming, while China went into lock-down within 21 days, the UK and many other countries only went into lock-down 2 to 3 months after the initial discovery of COVID-19, WHY? [China are now seeing a huge reduction in new cases and deaths, while the rest of the world's cases including the USA are spiralling upwards. China's reduction was because of the speed and effectiveness of their own countries internal lock-down.] I would suggest that the slowness of the rest of the world to act was due to their economies being more important at that stage than having a lock-down. Wealth over health scenario. Thankfully, this approach of wealth first has ended for the time being.

In a report released late last month, the World Health Organisation (WHO) congratulated China on a "unique and unprecedented public health response [that] reversed the escalating case."

Why have the developed countries of the world been so late in their lock-downs was it:

- Ignorance? Or

- Wealth prosperity? Or

- Unequivocal thinking that they are invincible, after all that's what Trump believed in?

What we can be sure of: The speed of the developed world's lock-down was an abysmal effort and represents the same effort that is being done to thwart climate change and that's not good or quick enough to avoid unnecessary illness and deaths.

Financial Cry for help, Vultures and an exit

As we come closer to an exit from the global pandemic, there have been cries for financial help from individuals, countries and businesses throughout the world. Let's hope that those cries are not deafened in countries attempts at regaining their own financial economies.

For example, in Spain, the Costa del Sol largely depends on a tourist trade and they are now warning of impending bankruptcy throughout the tourist industry. It is further believed that vulture funds could claim such businesses from the owners.

I hope and trust that all Governments will work together to ensure that the wealthy and stock market traders cannot profit from the misery of ordinary people and their businesses. As such, any exit plan must include substantial help and financial assistance to keep people in jobs and in business. Any pre and post exit plans must ensure that no one trading on shares can make a profit at the expense of this global pandemic. All Governments must stand together and block such scumbag tactics.

COVID-19 – Please stay safe

Can you remember what you were doing on Tuesday 31st December 2019? Were you getting ready for the New Year? Getting ready to go to bed or to party into the wee night hours?

While everyone was oblivious to the impending pandemic, the world continued with their daily rituals. Before midnight on the 31st December 2019 China reported a Pneumonia of an unknown cause that they detected in Wuhan, and subsequently they reported this to WHO's Country Office in China.

While you were celebrating the New Year Coronavirus was already partying and travelling to infect every other country in the world via foot, bicycle, car, bus, train, boat and aeroplane, perhaps even a few months earlier.

They call this version of the corona family of viruses COVID-19. And like the human population this virus wants to breed and populate, COVID-19 wants to live. I'm sure that humans would embrace this virus if it was a helpful virus, but like every other virus it infects humans in a way that can cause mild suffering to death. While COVID-19's effect on humans can be mild, those who are elderly or with underlying health issues could pay an ill-fated price of their life.

Now the search is on to find some sort of vaccine that can limit what the virus can do. Researchers and scientific teams are trying to understand COVID-19 so they can limit the dangers of contracting this virus. The world has come together in its efforts to halt this killing machine. But we all need to work together by self-isolating, practising social distancing and when feeling under the weather staying at home. Only go to the hospital or doctors if it is an emergency.

Health workers could be thought of being in the front line, however with this virus there is no front line, everyone has the potential to become infected. Therefore, every other person who works in essential services to ensure that the majority of the public have food, medicine, heating, maintenance, childcare, waste collection, street cleaning and so forth are doing a fantastic job. The list of essential workers is staggering, too many to list here. They are all putting their family's lives at risk of contracting COVID-19 so that our society continues to function.

Essential workers ensure that some sort of infrastructure continues for everyone.
The world says their deepest thanks to ALL essential workers and to those abiding by the rules.

- ALL essential workers are everyone's heroes. You might notice I put the word 'ALL', it is not just our NHS staff that's putting their life's in danger, but every person who is working and in contact with the public is at risk. My daughter works in an essential shop, she is surrounded by around 500 to 1,000 customers per day. My daughter has no protective garments as the NHS have, therefore she and the many others in similar positions of essential services are on the front line. So please spare a moment and remember all the people who are working to keep society with the ability to carry on living.

- Try and do you're shopping once per week and avoid stockpiling, only buy what you need and no more.

- To everyone else who are listening to the requests to remain at home and self-isolate, well done. You are ensuring that the health service has fewer cases and emergencies to deal with. I read a story about a Hasidic Jewish rabbi's funeral in Brooklyn, where hundreds of people were on the streets in extreme close proximity to each other and other members of the public. While we pay our condolences to the dead, we cannot allow any religion that thinks they can do what they want to do so. They too will abide by the same rules as most of the population, their religion should not offer them more rights than the ordinary person. It's just not on at all.

- If everyone plays their part as a unified team then we can all get through this together, quicker and safer.

- It was announced that a tiger in New York has tested positive for COVID-19, however there is no factual evidence that animals can infect humans. Furthermore, National Geographical has suggested that with the number of COVID-19 cases around the world if pets were an issue towards infection, then it would have been clear by now. However, I would suggest that you practice 'pet social distancing,' meaning when you are out with your pet, make sure your pet stays away from other people's pets.

Here are links to 2 interesting reports

The first is about how the coronavirus attacks the brain.

https://elemental.medium.com/coronavirus-might-attack-the-brain-too-21ea92a39c04

What makes COVID-19 unique?

https://medium.com/medical-myths-and-models/what-makes-the-novel-coronavirus-so-contagious-e677e825c566

Symptoms

CDC - https://qrs.ly/djbcy0k

Reported illnesses have ranged from mild symptoms to severe illness and death for confirmed coronavirus disease 2019 (COVID-19) cases. I'm sure when Boris Johnson gets back to work he will let us all know what the symptoms of his case were.

The following symptoms may appear 2-14 days after exposure.*

- Fever, Cough

- Shortness of breath

- Possibly a loss of smell

- Possibly a lack of taste

- Persistent pain in the chest

- Symptoms like a winter flu

*This is based on what has been seen previously as the incubation period of MERS-CoV viruses.

If you develop warning signs of having COVID-19 get medical attention immediately. Emergency warning signs include*:

- Difficulty breathing or shortness of breath

- Persistent pain or pressure in the chest

- New mental confusion, fatigue or inability to rouse

- Bluish lips or face [This shows a lack of Oxygen]

*This list is not all inclusive. Please consult your medical provider for any other symptoms that are severe or concerning.

Precautions

If you take the following precautions, you can limit the risk to yourself and others.

- Maintain good health, exercise and eat healthy

- Carry out all the health recommendations, like washing your hands REGULARLY, staying home if you are feeling sick, coughing or sneezing.

- Sneeze and cough into a tissue then bin it.

    - If you don't have a tissue then cough or sneeze into your arm and not into your hands.

    - Clean the clothes on your arm ASAP.

    - Empty your inside bin regular

- Avoiding close proximity to other people

- Make sure you clean your mobile phone regular, touching your dirty phone after washing your hands will have minor effect. Same applies to computer keyboards, games consoles, stair banisters, door handles etc.

- Avoid direct contact and maintain a distance from people who are more vulnerable to catching a virus.

- Clean surfaces regularly, that includes shopping baskets, shop shelves, floors and door handles to name only a few.

- Change your clothes and shower after returning from work or shopping

- Don't touch your eyes, mouth, nose or ears without thoroughly washing your hands first. Get out of the habit of touching your face, nose, mouth and ears.

I went to a local shopping centre just before they announced the lockdown. There was no hand sanitiser entering the building, nor was there any at the entrances to any of the shops within this building. Now most shopping centres are closed unless they have shops supplying essential goods to the public. Now most shops are providing hand and basket/trolley sanitiser as a prerequisite.

It's now May and some business that closed (UK), such as toy shops, builders merchants, paint shops etc. have reopened to supply products. However, to combat infection these stores request that you order in advance or know what you require, as they do not allow you entrance. You must que and their doorway and staff get you the products.

Another method to reduce infections is for food services to become home delivery, similar to take away food orders. Those that do not have access to Internet or the facility to order online would need further help.

Without a doubt the landscape of our current existence is about to change and possibly be redefined on how we do business in the future.

Make your own list of precautions, as the VIRUS knowledge develops so too will the need for extra precautions and methods to keep you safe.

The most important thing that you can do, is gain knowledge from reputable sources and recheck that information. Education sets you free. However, as you have seen on national news, even the president of the United States of America Donald Trump can give misleading and dangerous information. So don't take one person's viewpoint. Sometimes Trump can be correct, there is a lot of fake news out there, think out of the box for your own safety.

Testing people is one crutch to stop infections from spreading. The number of cases being officially announced is drastically short on what the real number could be if they carried mass testing out. Hence, the world calls on you to: "Stay at Home, only one person goes shopping, and maintain social distancing when shopping, working or exercising." That is not an infringement of your freedom. It's purely saving lives.

Where and when did the Virus Originate?

COVID-19 is a strain from the Coronavirus family of viruses. Some are less-severe, such as the common cold, and others develop into more severe disease such as Middle East respiratory syndrome (MERS) and Severe Acute Respiratory Syndrome (SARS) coronavirus.

On 31 December 2019, the World Health Organisation (WHO) where informed of a cluster of cases of pneumonia of unknown cause detected in Wuhan City, Hubei Province, China. [Extract and Source gov.uk]

On 1st January 2020, the city's Huanan Seafood Wholesale Market was shut down in China

On 12 January 2020 they announced that they had identified a novel coronavirus in human samples, and that initial analysis of this viruses genetic sequences suggested that this caused the outbreak. We refer this virus as SARS-CoV-2, and the associated disease as COVID-19 [Extract and Source gov.uk]

On 21st January 2020, the USA had its first case of COVID-19

On 23rd January 2020 China went into a FULL lock-down

On 11 February 2020, WHO announced a name for the unknown coronavirus disease, COVID-19? [Extract and Source Gov.uk]

On 21st February 2020 Italy went into lock-down

On 13th March Ireland went into lock-down with further restrictions being made on travel on 27th March

On 23rd March 2020 the UK went into lock-down.

The lack of speed in countries lock-downs is the true vehicle on how the virus spread. Especially the lack of halting international travel sooner than what the world did.

Source of Transmission

The source of the outbreak has yet to be determined but investigations are ongoing. Preliminary investigations identified environmental samples positive for SARS-CoV-2 in the Seafood Wholesale Market in Wuhan City, however some laboratory-confirmed patients did not report visiting this market.

Although evidence is still emerging, information to date shows human-to-human transmission is occurring. Precautions to prevent human-to-human transmission are appropriate for both suspected and confirmed cases (see infection prevention and control guidance).

We do not know the routes of transmission of COVID-19; however, other coronaviruses are mainly transmitted by large respiratory droplets and direct or indirect contact with infected secretions. Besides respiratory secretions, they have detected other coronaviruses in blood, faeces and urine.

Under certain circumstances, airborne transmission of other coronaviruses is thought to have occurred via unprotected exposure to aerosols of respiratory secretions and sometimes faecal material. [Extract and Source gov.uk]

Link to World Health Organisation (WHO) Interim Notice: Scan the QR image below and this will load a pdf document.

https://qrs.ly/axbcxzh

Clinical Features

Initial clinical findings from patients to date have been shared by China and WHO. Fever, cough or chest tightness, and dyspnoea are the major symptoms reported. While most patients have a mild illness, severe cases are also being reported, some of whom require intensive care.

We may expect a variety of abnormalities on chest radiographs, but bilateral lung infiltrates appear to be common (similar to what we see with other types of viral pneumonia). [Extract and Source gov.uk]

Who does it affect the most?

At present the virus seems to attack and be most dangerous for:

- The elderly and those over 60

- Anyone young or old with a lower immune system

- Those will other underlining health issues like heart disease, cancer, and smokers. It proves smoking reduces immunity (But it keeps flies and mosquito's away, it's true but I was being sarcastic)

Children are less affected by the virus but can be carriers of the virus without showing any warning signs. Therefore, some suggest to limit exposure to the elderly by both children and adults while the virus is on a rampage around the world. But make sure that any elderly person in your family or area knows that you will do their shopping and leave it at the door for them. Keep in touch with vulnerable groups of people, do not leave them to their own means. They need human contact as well via talking, joking and sharing conversations. At a time like this loneliness can be a killer.

Boris Johnson said, *"Things like closing schools and stopping big gatherings don't work as well perhaps as people think in stopping the spread,"* Why?

UPDATE: Turnaround by British Government: They have now

closed schools and have put the country in lock-down. Herd immunity was always a disastrous decision, as we don't know enough about this virus to allow the mass of public to become infected. And you do not need a medical degree to work that one out Mr. B. Johnson. Herd immunity for an unknown virus to which little is known is inaccurate and dangerous medical advice. Perhaps later on it could be expert advice, but not at present.

The Lock-down worked for China. As at 19th March recent cases and deaths in china have dramatically slowed down all because of their swift lock-down. Johnson and the conservative Government were initially only concerned with wealth generation and not health generation, closing businesses affects economic growth.

Italy, put its country on lock-down to avoid the virus spread despite the economic downturn it will face.

It's like the catholic, the protestant and the Muslim debating god and religion. Sometimes you will get nowhere fast while the world around us perishes into a plume of mind boggling endless debate on whose god or religion is the worthiest. Or an even better analogy, visualise the worlds Government representatives at the last COP25 conference, lots of talk...but no action on reduction of fossil fuel emission, only talk and more talk and a move for more talk at the next COP26 meeting in Glasgow in 2020. And now there is a good chance COP26 will be postponed because of COVID-19.

Can you imagine if countries were to talk and postpone any Coronavirus action? Ops! That's another million dead.

But yet our Governments forget about the millions that are dying every year via cancer and pollution. Where is the same emergency for those people dying because of pollution from oil, coal, gas production, tobacco use & production, plastic manufacturing etc.? Why are these cancerous industries allowed to continue, WHY?

How did it spread?

Common sense simplistic example: 1st infected person, they go to a shop to buy some groceries (that's 1 person infected), they sit in a restaurant (that's 1 waiter infected), they get onto a packed bus (that's 4 passengers infected), they get off the bus and go to the airport passing many people (that's 20 more infected), on the aircraft (30 more passengers are infected), when the infected people arrive at their destination or in another country they now begin to spread the disease as they go about their travels. Have you got the picture yet?

The above represents the journey of the 1st infected person for one day. Now take the above and do the same one day journey for each person who has been infected from the 1st person. Now the infected people move around all week. The infection has now become international, it's now a pandemic. We have all seen the movies, yet Governments moved painfully slow to halt the spread of COVID-19

Large movement hubs like airports, train stations, bus stations, boat terminals, shopping centres, schools, universities, doctors surgeries, hospitals, large-scale events and so forth where everyone are in close proximity ensures that the virus will spread at exponential rates.

The instant they announced the virus in China, the world should have been in immediate lock-down, and not 2, or 3 months later. Any lock-down was only at its most effective if done at the same time as China's lock-down.

Neither can you blame China for this outbreak, the USA president should be ashamed of himself for calling it a Chinese virus. In fact all of his aids and Republican Party should be downright ashamed when they stood by him without changing their facial expressions when he announced that message. Shame on you... this demonstrates that Trump's administration are the parasites of the American people. And they do not deserve or have the right or respect to be in power.

A lack of hygiene both personal and public helps spread the virus. Lack of deep cleans within traffic hubs, public places, and businesses aids the transmission of the virus. At home you could practice a daily ritual of cleaning handles, surfaces, shoes, floor, counters, furniture, try to make your home coronavirus free. As a family when I return with the shopping I wipe all the packaging down with an antibacterial wipe before it enters our home.

The virus wants to live, it has a job to be done, and the virus takes no prisoners. In its current form it will attempt to claim the life of any person who is in the vulnerability domain. Most deaths from COVID-19 is currently from vulnerable groups of people. But evolution could change the virus to become more dangerous to other non-vulnerable people. Likewise the flu, climate change and pollution infect the vulnerable and non-vulnerable. How many healthy people do you know that have contracted the flu or cancer and have subsequently died? This is not a natural death, its murder by your Government, they are the ones guilty of allowing corporations to do what they want. The business model is wealth before Health.

Oil, coal and tobacco related illness spread as the demand for these products increase. To make things worse, products are manufactured in countries that are manipulated via cheap labour and raw materials to serve a growing demand in developed countries. Production of oil, coal, gas and tobacco products became an everyday requirement.

Since 1912 scientists warned of the dangers to your health and our planet through the continued use of fossil fuels. But these big businesses are too ingrained into our fabric and economic system that Governments and Politician's lack any real gumption to do the right thing and create a lock-down to halt their production. Because wealth and a financial economy comes first over people's health and welfare.

Incubation Period

The "incubation period" means the time between catching the virus and beginning to have symptoms of the disease. Most estimates of the incubation period for COVID-19 range from 1 to 14 days, most commonly around five days. They will update these estimates as more data become available. [Extract and Source from WHO]

How long can the virus Live on surfaces?

It is uncertain how long the virus that causes COVID-19 survives on surfaces. But it seems to be similar to other coronaviruses. Studies suggest that coronaviruses (including preliminary information on the COVID-19 virus) may persist on surfaces for a few hours or up to several days. This may vary under different conditions (e.g. type of surface, temperature or humidity of the environment).

If you think a surface may be infected, clean it with simple disinfectant to kill the virus and protect yourself and others. Clean your hands with an alcohol-based hand rub or wash them with soap and water. Avoid touching your eyes, mouth, or nose. [Extract and Source from WHO]

Scan the QR image below to view a report by the BBC science team on how long the virus can stay alive on surfaces

https://qrs.ly/6rbe0z9

Is there anything I should NOT do?

The following measures ARE NOT effective against COVID-2019 and can be harmful:

- Smoking

- Wearing multiple masks

- Taking antibiotics (See question 10 "Are there any medicines of therapies that can prevent or cure COVID-19? Scan code to go to q10 and others")

- Do not take anti-inflammatory pain tablets. Take paracetamol instead, (See medications below)

If you have **fever, cough and difficulty breathing seek medical care early to reduce the risk of developing a more severe infection** and be sure to share your recent travel history with your health care provider. [Extract and Source from WHO]

For other frequent asked questions scan the QR image below to go to the WHO FAQ.

https://qrs.ly/qmbcy0h

Medications to relieve symptoms

The French Government reported that "grave adverse effects" are linked to the use of non-steroidal anti-inflammatory drugs (NSAID). Frances health Minister Olivier Veran, tweeted that *"taking anti-inflammatory drugs (ibuprofen, cortisone...) could be an aggravating factor of the COVID-19 infection. If you have a fever, take paracetamol. If you are already on anti-inflammatory drugs or in doubt, ask your doctor for advice."*

Some health experts throughout the world have stated that it is too soon because of the lack of scientific evidence suggesting any possible links between ibuprofen and adverse effects of coronavirus.

Paracetamol has been cited as better than anti-inflammatory drugs on this Covid occasion as the safer option. However, check with your doctor before making any decision, they are the ones being kept up-to-date with coronavirus updates.

GET PROPER MEDICAL ADVICE, and not from twitter, Facebook or posts by 'granny doctor or Donald Trump'

Travel Advice

Below is a link to the UK Government Coronavirus travel advice. However, it would be advisable to check your own countries website for details. Airports and sea terminals have begun to either cancel or reduce transportation to other countries, and even movement within a country. Some airlines have announced that they will begin flights as from mid-June 2020.

News-update: All but essential travel has been stopped in many countries throughout the world.

It is the advice of many countries to travel only if necessary.

The UK Government has issued the following statement regarding cruise holidays: *"If you are planning to go on a cruise, be aware a COVID-19 outbreak on board is possible, and your travel may be disrupted... If you are aged 70 and over, or if you have underlying health conditions, we advise you against cruise ship travel at this time."*

Entry restrictions: *"Many countries and territories have introduced screening measures (temperature checks and health/travel questions) and entry restrictions at border crossings and transport hubs... If you have recently been in a country affected by the virus you may need to be quarantined, or you may not be allowed to enter or travel through a third country."* As at 24th March many countries have stopped all flights apart from essential service flights.

When travel does begin, you should still take precautions. The end of COVID-19 does not imply ending common sense. You never know we might even slow down the flu virus.

https://qrs.ly/xcbd1ev

Travel Advice after Lockdown

Ryanair have announced that they will fly 1,000 daily flights from 1st July 2020 pending Government restrictions being lifted. They have even produced a video explaining their extra measures and how they will keep you safe. It will also be subject to other countries lifting their restrictions and allowing flights in.

But wait for it…

- You will be asked to wear masks at the airport and on Ryanair aircraft. They did not say who will provide these masks? But we all know Ryanair, so I'm sure they will sell masks? Or will the airport provide masks?

- They are asking you to keep a safe social distance, no mention of it being mandatory. Bearing in mind if you follow Ryanair's previous boarding policy, it was get on as fast as you can so they can get in the air quicker. Will Ryanair and airports be allowing a longer boarding time?

- They are asking you to take your own temperature before you leave home. Plus the airport MIGHT do a temperature check. Are they going to trust people's word on temperature checks?

- Foremost people can still carry the virus and show no signs of any temperature increase. And there is still a possibility they could be able to transmit the virus to you, regardless of wearing a mask or not. Only testing will truly identify who has the virus.

- Clean and disinfect the aircraft once per day with super 24 hour disinfectant. That's a lame excuse, long before the last flight of the day for that aircraft your arse would have totally wiped away all disinfectant on that seat. All flights should be disinfected at the end of every flight, but that would delay Ryanair's flights and cost more money. I would need to see testing proof that demonstrated how long the disinfected items stayed disinfected after hundreds if not thousands of touches, rubbing and movement over these surfaces.

- Ryanair are encouraging people to buy fast track and priority boarding so that the ques will be less. If everyone buys priority and fast track, there will still be a que, and Ryanair would have more income. It is also legalised segregation through a person's income levels. If you have more money you better health protection boarding.

Ryanair have even enlisted a Biochemistry and Immunology celebrity professor Luke O'Neil from TCD to inform you that a mask will catch 95% of the virus been excreted via mouth and nose. However, in February 2020 Mr O'Neil stated that wearing a mask was only effective if you had the virus, and if you are healthy and your immune system is good, then you will be ok.

What about infection from tears (low, they reckon only around 1% to 3% infection rate?)

However, an infected person can release the virus into the air by coughing, sneezing or talking, these virus particles can then enter via your eyes, mouth or nose.

The World Health Organisation has stated the following about masks, they also recommend medical masks as being the most effective.

- *If you are healthy, you only need to wear a mask if you are taking care of a person with COVID-19.*
- *Wear a mask if you are coughing or sneezing.*
- *Masks are effective only when used in combination with frequent hand-cleaning with alcohol-based hand rub or soap and water.*
- *If you wear a mask, then you must know how to use it and dispose of it properly.*
- *Replace the mask with a new one as soon as it is damp and do not re-use single-use masks. (How will you do that safely on an aircraft?)*

The World Health Organisation has made a recent update in line with the easing of the lock-downs and now recommends that the wearing of masks should become mandatory when travelling and in shops.

Air companies like many other businesses are haemorrhaging money therefore they are overly keen to get into the air with as many passengers as their planes will hold. Hotels and holiday resorts are equally desperate to open for business. Plus Governments don't want to keep bailing businesses and individuals out of this pandemic of a financial problem. The UK Government have so far provided Jet2 with over £400 million in aid.

Moreover, I believe that reducing the lockdown because of the economy is the incorrect attitude to take. I further believe that if transportation hubs and onward/inward travels do not have effective and tough legislation, then this could be the creation of a second major spike in the viruses' future of transmission around the globe. Governments cannot rely on companies to introduce their own rules. Governments need to be the leaders and tell companies what the mandatory rules are. Just now it's a free for all.

The sadness is money is driving us out of lockdown sooner than what it should be. O'Leary and Ryanair shareholders don't want to lose the wealth that they have built up. We need to question the motives behind the rich before we can accept their word. History has shown that the spread and subsequent world transmission of the virus was attained by transportation between countries. It would also be safe to assume that if we allow international travel on the scale as before (meaning full flights, full airports etc.) then it is possible that people with no signs of being infected could infect others at any transportation hub. (Flights, buses, subways, trains, boats etc.)

I further believe that virus testing should be mandatory for all exits and entrances at every border. However, that would slow everything down but at least it would be safer albeit at a greater cost. It's a tough decision to make, but the right decision should be Health before wealth. Or are we now entering the phase of deaths to be termed collateral damage for wealth creation of others?

Prevention Future Solutions

- Provide health education and help to countries towards good health and hygiene and the health risks from markets who sell dead and live food. This creates a heightened risk of 'virus jumping' from animals to humans. This is directly because of hygiene standards becoming difficult to maintain when animals are butchered next to live animals. Another factor is the density of people and animals crammed into these markets, this facilitates and allows any disease to spread between species.

- China and India have enormous populations that require feeding and suitable and hygienic planning needs to be factored to facilitate healthy living standards, ending poverty would aid that development, and would help stop pollution and viruses from spreading.

- Stop keeping animals in confined spaces like battery hens, this increases the risk of infections spreading rapidly.

- Dangerous cooking habits and eating some animals can lead to the spread of diseases and hence the evolution of diseases from animal to human. Use and develop other sustainable sources such as plant-based foods. Not only would you be healthier but you would be helping our planet.

- It could carry testing out at transportation hubs prior to leaving a country

- Faster lock-down of towns, cities and countries after a virus outbreak.

- International financial help for countries and people during and after a lock-down

- Health to come first over wealth.

- Tele-conferencing can take place as an alternative to meetings. As was with a recent sports event. No public only the players, everyone else watched from home.

- Make any future travel to adhere to the social distancing that means that transport (Flights, trains, planes etc.) and transportation hubs (airports, sea, bus and train terminals)cannot be jammed packed as previously in the past.

We are already seeing an increase of businesses in the UK and Ireland creating working from home solutions. Could this become the new normal? From an environmental impact viewpoint, it would mean fewer co2 emissions. Large office buildings would no longer be required and it would achieve savings on energy. Demolish these buildings and erect solar energy facilities or create new greenways to trap co2.

Since the outbreak of Coronavirus pollution has dropped, but still not enough to make a lasting difference for our climate.

The campaign to halt the use of fossil fuels must continue. If countries are now willing to lock-down cities and countries over COVID-19, then we must surly have the mentality to make drastic changes to save humanity from climate cancer, because that has the possibility to kill all of us.

China's resurgence of the virus

While China has now been relatively free from fresh cases and deaths. May is seeing a new small resurgence of coronavirus within China. So this implies while the Chinese lock-down was far superior to the wests, the west would expect a resurgence on a larger scale to that of China's resurgence of the virus.

All exit plans must include a safe distancing and reduced numbers in work, schools, hotels, restaurants, production lines, factories, shops, transportation and hospitals, this list is not exhaustible. But the point I'm making is that any exit must be crystal clear, and it should not be business as usual.

Statistics and
Should Coronavirus COVID-19 be taken seriously?
COVID-19 as at 29th March 2020, China has:

81,439	Case's
3,300	Deaths
75,448	Total recovered
2,691	Active Cases

As at 6th April 2020, China had reported: 81,708 cases and 3,331 deaths

From the statistics above china has a death rate of 4% of cases reported. The UK has a death rate of 4.8% of cases reported. However, Italy has a staggering death rate of 10.8% of cases reported. However, statistics can mislead, in this case because of the lack of population testing and hence many thousands more cases might not of been reported.

It is important that everyone takes care and to limit the spread of this virus by self-isolating and maintaining a social distance and going out only when necessary.

- **Of course COVID-19 should be taken seriously.** And everyone that can should be self-isolating. However key workers will carry on working, while ensuring taking steps to remain safe. There will be many others working from home

- You should also take the flu virus seriously,

- The climate emergency should be taken seriously,

- And earth's pollution definitely should be taken seriously.

- COVID-19 is affecting the elderly with underling health issues and vulnerable children and adults. Therefore, everyone in these groups should self-isolate. We should help the vulnerable while following health guidance on doing this.

- COVID-19 is the first new virus pandemic that is spreading throughout the world and is killing people. But in reality cancer is a larger pandemic. The number of cancer deaths is growing each year. The more our atmosphere becomes polluted the more that people will become infected with cancer.

- The USA have predicted that 606,520 people will die from cancer in 2020. Derived from pollution, fossil fuel emissions, tobacco smoking (production & emissions), and unhealthy eating.

Scan Image below to watch a video describing the Coronavirus (WHO)

https://qrs.ly/enbcxzf

Scan QR image to go to the NHS website for further info on Coronavirus COVID-19

https://qrs.ly/c1bcxyt

I believe that the COVID-19 outbreak and the world's response, could be viewed as a mini dress rehearsal for what will happen when our climate disaster kicks in.

COVID-19 and the world's response is only a ripple in the ocean to what will actually occur in ten to thirty years' time if we don't stop climate change now. Economies of the world could become bankrupt, panic and civil riots could break out in a magnitude never witnessed before.

But there is HOPE, if the world joins together and makes a cohesive action plan with immediate action to address three major problems then we stand a chance of creating a glorious future for our children and the next generations. (1. Fossil fuel and Pollution elimination-land-oceans-atmosphere, 2. Sustainable energy, food & environment model and 3. Health & equality before wealth & inequality)

For those that live in robust and developed countries please spare thoughts for other less financially robust countries who will suffer economically from the results of coronavirus, more than what you can imagine. I hope that our Governments help these countries and their populations without any delay.

And I hope our Governments stand by their own people and help immediately and when necessary. (Time will surely tell on that) **UPDATE:** The UK Government have announced a £350 Billion package to help the public and businesses. The USA have announced financial packages to help corporations. I hope that countries will rally together and help other countries and their populations.

In a nutshell, coronavirus [the COVID-19 strain] is affecting 210 countries and territories around the world and 2 cruise ships.

As at 29th of March 2020 there have been 669,102 COVID-19 cases worldwide and 31,068 deaths. As at 10th April 2020 there have been 1,677,286 cases and 101,577 deaths.

However, the number of cases and deaths in China have slowed down dramatically since 17th March 2020. For the last few days China has reported as little as 30 to 90 new cases and 8 deaths per day. However Italy's, Spain's and France's deaths and cases are soaring.

Statistic's as at 23rd, 26th, 29th March, 10th April and 21st December 2020

Country	Cases	Deaths	Population Estimated at 2020
China: (23rd)	81,093	3,270	
(26th)	81,285	3,287	1,439,323,776
(29th)	81,439	3,300	
(10/4)	81,907	3,336	
(21/12)	86,852	4,634	
Italy: (23rd)	63,927	6,077	
(26th)	74,386	7,503	60,461,826
(29th)	92,472	10,023	
(10/4)	143,626	18,279	
(21/12)	1,964,054	69,214	
Iran: (23rd)	23,049	1,812	
(26th)	29,406	2,234	83,992,949
(29th)	35,408	2,517	
(10/4)	68,192	4,232	
(21/12)	1,164,535	53,816	
Spain: (23rd)	33,089	2,207	
(26th)	56,188	4,089	46,754,778
(29th)	73,235	5,982	
(10/4)	157,022	15,843	
(21/12)	1,830,110	49,260	
USA (23rd)	42,484	517	
(26th)	68,594	1,038	331,002,651
(29th)	123,781	2,229	
(10/4)	475,659	17,838	
(21/12)	18,425,166	326,312	
UK: (23rd)	6,650	335	
(26th)	9,539	465	67,886,011
(29th)	17,089	1,019	
(10/4)	65,077	7,978	
(21/12)	2,073,511	67616	
Ireland:(23rd)	1,125	6	
(26th)	1,564	9	4,937,786
(29th)	2,415	36	
(10/4)	6,574	263	
(21/12)	80,267	2,158	

The table was created by the author from data sourced from '"WHO' and 'Worldometers.info'.
As at 21/12/20: USA, India, Brazil, Russia, France and UK are the top 6 countries with the most infections.

In the 17 day reporting period (March to April 2020) as shown in the table above the number of cases in the USA has increased by 11 times. In the subsequent eight months up to 21st December 2020, the cases have again multiplied by 38.8 times. Are these dramatic increases directly due to Trump and his administration's original denial on coronavirus or indeed his refute of social distancing? And Trump made blatantly stupid remarks to encourage people not to comply, such as, "Are you wearing a mask and his many mass gatherings with no social distancing and no masks. Or did Trump not want a lock-down because it could affect his own personal businesses and wealth? Or was it pressure from large corporations re political and economic reasons? But the likely answer was all of those. You the American people can be the judge and Jury on that one.

% Death Rate based on Reported Cases vs Number of Deaths
As at 21st December 2020

USA	1.8%
India	1.5%
Brazil	2.6%
Russia	1.8%
France	2.5%
UK	3.3%
Italy	3.5%
Spain	2.7%
Iran	4.6%
China	5.3%
Ireland	2.7%

The above death rate percentages statistics should be read with precaution. Why?

1) Reported figures could be incorrect or reported falsely
2) The higher the number of cases could imply that more non

vulnerable people are catching Covid and as such they are not dying

3) The death rate percentage could be misleading as many who recover could have went through severe pain or near death experiences. As such this is not recorded in above percentages. The reason I mention this, some people will look at these percentages as low and worth the risk. However, just like a severe accident that you recover from you would not want to go through a severe bout of Covid. This information has sadly been missed out by hospital or home records. The main reason I state this, is if people become complacent then cases will rise dramatically, and hospitals could become inundated to a degree that they can't function correctly, and that in turn puts more people at risk to die.

Covid acts swiftly to infect you therefore you can become sick extremely quick. That puts a strain on medical health professionals and their ability to deal with other life threatening illness like cancer and other day to day admittances at hospitals.

Since they announced the outbreak in December 2019, China's cases and deaths have slowed down considerably. Was this because of their proactive lock-down measures? It took USA and most other countries up to 3 months before they locked down? And even now, countries are having many small separate and un-coordinated lockdowns.

In order for any short term lockdown to be effective, it must be a worldwide event. But alas, nine months later and the world's leaders still do not have a clue.

There is also a consensus that perhaps COVID-19 was around and causing infection well before December 2019.

There are many conspiracy theories, but I'm not going to give any of these any credence at this point. Moreover, pharmaceutical companies should not be allowed to profiteer off the backs of this pandemic. If they are allowed to do so then this will be a tragedy towards humanity. Neither should they be allowed to hike wages or receive excessive bonuses in order to reduce profits, this should be taken as treason if they do.

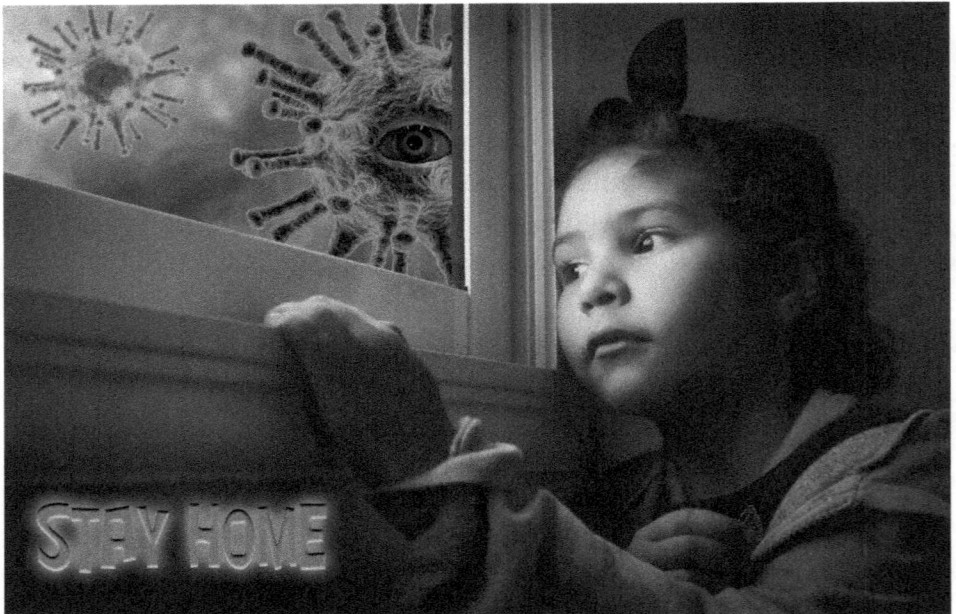

Should we suffer and Die - COVID-19 and Climate Cancer?

The Coronavirus has created **havoc** amongst the world's population. It has become the most discussed and news reported topic on the day's agenda throughout the world. You can't go a second without some news flash or thought entering your neuro-pathways on its journey to enlighten or terrify your brain on the effects of COVID-19.

People are concerned, school children and adults are talking about their fears. Because it's real, it's in the news and its happening, right now. People don't want to die. But this is the 'double edge sword mentality.' Pollution, is real and has been scientifically proved to cause over 1 million cancer deaths per year. Climate cancer is killing people every day on a massive scale, most people know someone who has died from cancer. I have friends and family that died from cancer.

What's amazing is the empathy, scale and 'action plan' to halt the COVID-19 pandemic as compared to the world's **miserable attempt** at stopping climate change and the deaths that occur directly from Government's failure to halt climate change.

Sure we have cancer charities and many groups fighting this illness. But the crux and most important point is while we are all fighting this horrific cancer disease, we let the perpetrators of its creation carry on to infect millions more people every single year.

Oil companies, coal plants, tobacco companies, plastic manufacturing, gold mining, fracking, breweries, and many more industries are all getting away with murdering humans, animals, and now the planet itself is in genuine danger. And our Governments allow this to happen, many Politician's and Governments are the 'mouth pieces' of the oil, coal, gas, plastics and tobacco giants. These companies fund Politician's campaigns for re-election and they therefore help shape Government policies. This is not right! And we must stop this practice.

The USA president Trump and his administration are the backers of these polluters. The American people need to do the right thing, remove Trump and the Republicans from power.

Today, I drove behind a double-decker bus [Driving a fossil fuel car that emits co2 into the air, feeling as guilty as hell. But I like many others needed my car that day to complete my daily tasks within an approved time frame, school to work to school to shopping... no car = no work, no school, no food, catch-22 situation. Yet our Governments are doing little to make electric cars available for the majority of people at an affordable price. Nor are they providing a green public transportation system that allows people to complete their journeys without the need of private transport and within an acceptable time frame.

Like always the little people will get the scraps from the rich. But only this time it will be too late for our climate and our health.

Back to my bus story, on the back of this double-decker bus was a full advert displaying a bottle of beer and a glass of beer. After overtaking the bus I discovered it was full of school children. Yep, that's our marketing and advertising board for you, encouraging our children to drink. They banned smoking adverts, alcohol adverts should be barred, but it's like the climate emergency, banning adverts would be a financial loss for advertisers and breweries, plus remember the Government make a considerable revenue from alcohol & tobacco taxes. So Governments allow most of the population to suffer and die so that big business and their shareholders can make loads of dosh while maintaining our economies. Under the current world's economies, wealth creation comes first before Health creation. That is a travesty for humanity.

That's what you call the "Suffer and Die from big business Cancer link." Profits are before people, they allow people to suffer so that the rich can get richer, while big business, Governments and education promise you the same chance of wealth creation. But it's a false dream. You work even harder in your attempts to achieve financial stardom. But in reality you suffer so they can profit from your misery. You were NOT born into this world to serve anyone.

Perhaps coronavirus will give the world a break from their fast paced every day ritual of work and sleep mentality? Perhaps people can slow down for a month or so and recuperate and really think and research what these big businesses and lack of Government action are doing to your health?

Many people are suffering from anxiety. **Being coup up inside could affect the mentality of people.** Children need contact with their friends. A lock-down will affect people in ways that have not been seen before. This is a new world being born right in front of us.

I hope social workers are still working and looking after the interests of vulnerable children, women and men. This lock-down could intensify problems for those vulnerable or indeed those living within homes of adversity. Therefore it is a necessity that social workers and the Government are being proactive and are doing their part in ensuring the safety of vulnerable children and others. Social workers are an essential service and should be working towards addressing the needs of these groups of people.

After the pandemic passes we could find that many people will need support both mentally and financially to help them cope with the COVID-19 aftermath.

We must be mindful of the impact of a lock-down on the mental health of everyone, we do not want to see an increase in mental health issues or suicides. As such Governments and the health service needs to be proactive in sorting this out sooner rather than later. Fix it now and not after the event.

COVID-19 Brings hope to our Climate and pollution

One thing for sure, the atmosphere is getting a breather in the form of a vast reduction in co2 and pollution emissions. Our air can actually breathe again.

Scan the image to watch the video on china's clear skies.

https://qrs.ly/5cbddgx

The following is an extract from The Telegraph newspaper regarding the worlds shutdown: **Blue skies, dolphins and clear canals in Venice – the beautiful side effects of the coronavirus pandemic** *"Swans in canals, dolphins at empty cruise ports and even wild boar in cobbled streets prove how fast nature can reclaim the world...It has to be said, Planet Earth would breathe a long sigh of relief if humans were to vanish. And temporarily, in many places, they have...Amid the unprecedented coronavirus global lock-down, scenes worthy of a Disney film have emerged; from swans gliding through the now-clear canals of Venice to blue skies over China where the air is usually choked with smog."*

Our air quality around the world is getting better, thanks to the Coronavirus outbreak.

Image above courtesy of NASA and European Space Agency (ESA)

The image below shows that pollution over Italy is decreasing rapidly. Picture below courtesy of Santiago Gasso.

Drastic reduction in pollution

Similar to China's reductions in pollution because of COVID-19, Italy is now seeing a dramatic reduction in pollution.

Nitrogen dioxide levels in the air above Italy's Po Valley decline as the country enters coronavirus ... [+] @CREACleanAir

Drastic reductions in pollution can only mean one thing for the world, and that's a safer and brighter future for all life forms on earth. Hopefully, a continued reduction in pollution will continue on the exit from lockdown.

One thing for sure climate justice cannot accept Governments utilising a Trojan horse in the guise of increasing pollution in their attempts to recover their economy.

Pollution has been reduced, it must stay that way for the sake of human kind's future. Money, wealth and an economy cannot come before the health of our planet.

Extract from the Director General of WHO

"Several countries have demonstrated that this virus can be suppressed and controlled....

1. *First, prepare and be ready.*

2. *Second, detect, protect and treat.*

3. *Third, reduce transmission.*

4. *Fourth, innovate and learn...*

And let's all look out for each other, because we need each other."
Source: Director of World Health Organisation (WHO.int)

Let's hope all the Governments follow this advice both for the COVID-19 pandemic and the climate change pandemic which is on course to alter history if we don't all do something radical to stop it.

Some Governments have reacted quickly in their attempt to try and limit the spread and reduce deaths arising from COVID-19. Italy for example is in total lock-down. Other countries are likely to follow suit as the virus spreads. **Why can't Government's act as quickly for the climate emergency?**

Some websites to check for information

https://www.who.int/

https://www.who.int/emergencies/diseases/novel-coronavirus-2019

Scam Alert:

https://www.who.int/about/communications/cyber-security

In the initial days supermarkets limited sales of some food and toilet paper because you have selfish people **stockpiling** and leaving the rest of the community without. What happened to compassion and thinking about each other?

The photographs below represent the start of the lock-down and now (May 2020)

Our health service workers are at the forefront of the sick and ensure that people are cared for. Our thanks and gratitude goes out to all the various services that are involved with helping people in this pandemic, including all the people on the front line ensuring that we have all the facilities available to us. Like, street cleaners, the cleansing departments, plumbers, joiners, and food manufacturers, farmers supplying our food, shops, ambulances, fire brigade, police, armed forces, lifeboats and rescue services. This list is not exhaustive. They are all the true heroes of the day.

Herd Immunity

If we review some death statistics, you have a far greater chance of being killed or seriously injured in a road traffic accident, or dying from the flu, or dying from cancer or if you are still around in 10 to 30 years dying because of climate cancer than dying from COVID-19. With that being said let's look at what Boris Johnson has suggested below in regard to Herd immunity.

"According to a recent ITV report, the British Government is reportedly hoping to reduce the impact of the virus by allowing it to, "pass through the entire population so that we acquire herd immunity" Source Independent Newspapers and ITV interview.

The Government's chief scientific adviser Sir Patrick Vallance has told Sky News that about 60% of people will need to become infected with coronavirus in order for the UK to enjoy "herd immunity." Scan the QR image below to see the Sky News Interview.

https://qrs.ly/6sbcxz4

Herd immunity initially suits the British Government and Trumps administration to a tee. If your Government were to utilise this technique, the economy would benefit over the lives of people. After all the Tory Government along with Trump stands for wealth creation and not Health creation. When it comes to the economy, wealth is first before Health. Little people are purely pawns in the equation that feeds the wealth creators.

Herein lays the foremost reason why the UK, USA and other Governments did not immediately go into lock-down. For purely financial reasons. However, with increasing pressure of rising cases and deaths around the world the policy changed to become a directive to limit the collateral damage to people's health and lives.

Moreover,

- This is why the climate disaster is not receiving adequate funding and major bureaucracy against any immediate action.

- That's why you have millions dying with cancer every year. Somehow the shift from stopping the cause of cancer became charity fundraising events to help find a cure for cancer. The major deterrent is starring us straight in the face, STOP FOSSIL FUEL production and its use and stop pollution. This is within the ability of every person on this planet. But wealth before health and our current financial economy stops the most obvious solution from happening.

Governments call your families deaths "collateral damage," as it burns fossil fuels and pollutes our atmosphere on its pathway towards a financial economy, where the rich get richer and the poorer get poorer. So much so it gets to a stage where it becomes difficult to fight against these tyrants. But fight we will, our children's future will come first before any Politician's manifesto.

The time is now, we need to vote ineffective Politician's out of office and replace them with people who will make a difference for people's health and the climate. Let's get climate justice and a destruction in using fossil fuels. A new breed of Politician's is demanded now, people who use common sense to make changes that are needed. Health should always come first over wealth.

There is always a 'but', but drastic change will need the support of every country and every person, we are all in this together. Climate cancer can be cured, but we need the support of everyone. Countries need to change from wealth creation to Health Creation and become a caring humanity.

On your death bed you will not be judged on your wealth but on your good deeds towards each other. We all know where Trump, dictators and others in a similar boat are going on their death. There are no accepted confessions on earth only viewable and humane actions will be your testament to any afterlife. How can a billionaire die in peace when their wealth could have stopped hunger, poverty and homelessness to name a few? How can a millionaire look at their wealth while others suffer in poor health because of poverty?

Donald Trump, USA President is IDIOT-1
And his virus statements demonstrates this status:

Ladies, Gentlemen, children and people of the world you know of COVID-19, I would like to introduce you to IDIOT-1.

IDIOT-1 is the president of the United States of America. Furthermore, Trump is incapable of accepting any blame for anything. He is a prime example of the most unsatisfactory person to be in a presidency, ever and not a role model for our children.

If you were to make similar remarks as he does then you would be prosecuted for slanderous, racist comments and false information. Trump and the USA Republican Party have well-earned this IDIOT-1 title for their downright stupidity and ignorance over many debates. However, Trump has exceeded his IDIOT-1 title for changing the name Coronavirus to be renamed as the 'Chinese Virus.' The latest crap from the president's mouth was to inject yourself with household disinfectants, to which he tried to backtrack from days later. However, the truth was watched by billions of people around the world. What is even worse he and his administration tried to weasel themselves out of any wrong doing. Scumbags!

https://qrs.ly/s1bdv62

https://qrs.ly/ogbdvjw

Trump is a savvy and brilliant businessman who can easily and psychologically twist and turn around words so that the public are brainwashed into thinking what he wants them to believe. As such he kept on insisting that the virus did come from China, and that he is right in what he says. That's what you call a twisting and manipulative president that deserves no respect whatsoever. It's a president that is psychosomatically abusing the people of his country.

That's like the old American slave labour colony days and I believe in some areas of the states it still exists. For example, if one shooter or pimp is black, then the suggestion and hence assumption that all Black people are shooters or pimps. That last statement is incorrect and racist. That's the mentality that the president of the United States is being allowed to similarly project in many situations and debates. This is not only scandalous but downright manipulative and disgraceful.

The American public need to vote for a young and energetic president that can take the USA into a new world where people's Health comes before that of wealth. And a president that will move forward with climate change in a manner never witnessed before, including the immediate halt of all fossil fuel production and its use. That type of leader would make 'America great again.' That type of leader would gain the worlds respect, that type of leadership would guarantee a fit place in their next life.

The need for ventilators, what a USA mess

*"The President of USA said today that governors should try to get things like respirators and masks on their own..."*Source: http://www.centerforhealthsecurity.org/

Is it me, is it us?

- Maybe it's me, perhaps I'm the Idiot?

- Are my morals are all wrong? Of course, we should agree to the financial economy being more important than the death of millions of people each year via pollution that our

Governments are allowing to happen on a daily basis.

- Of course, we are all the idiots.

Yes, I'm getting the picture now, it's becoming perfectly clear, and we are ALL the idiots. But wait, that's what they want you and me to believe. The fact that your child, mother, father, brother, sister, friend, uncle, aunt, grandmother, grandfather, husband, wife are contracting cancer and dying in painful circumstances **is proof that we are the idiots.**

We are all idiots when we stand by and let our Governments dictate to us that your child, or your mother, or your father's deaths are collateral damage. **Yep, that's collateral damage so that others can profit from their deaths.**

We are the idiots for allowing this to occur. When has money and wealth come before that of a person's life? Tell me, please tell me, WHEN?

If I informed Donald Trump that his children will die tomorrow from cancer. But if we stop fossil fuel production and pollution IMMEDIATELY they will live. **What would he choose?**

If I informed Boris Johnson that he could stop cancer virtual overnight and save millions of lives per year by halting fossil fuel use and production. **What would he choose?**

If I informed Governments around the world that if they choose Health Creation over Wealth Creation, they could eliminate cancer and the climate emergency and save millions of lives. **What would they choose?**

To our Politician's and leaders, imagine that you have a child, and your child is looking into your eyes with tears in their dying eyes. Mummy, Daddy the doctor told me if you stop polluting my town with co2... I will live. **What will you do?**

To our Politician's and leaders, imagine that your child is lying on the street with their last breath. An angel from above comes down and tells you that your child will live if you do one thing. That one thing is putting Human health and prosperity BEFORE that of Human Wealth and Financial prosperity. **What would you choose?**

Now look at yourself in the mirror and ask yourself **why you are allowing cancer and climate damage to continue?** We need to campaign our Governments with the same ferocity that we are fighting human cancer to end human and climate cancer.

Human Cancer is Climate Cancer…

Climate Cancer is the cause of Human Cancer…

They are both intrinsically linked

Jobs vs Pollution & Cancer

A plastics manufacturing company called Formosa was at the blunt of hundreds of civil rights and environmental lawsuits in the USA. Several of its employees became whistle-blowers because of the destruction that the plant and its chemicals were doing to the water and atmosphere. People were developing cancer. Their fellow workers intimidated and attacked those who became whistle blowers.

Now what does that tell you? It lets you know that having a job and earnings is more important than children dying with cancer. Being able to put food on the table for their family is more important than contracting cancer and other chemical related diseases.

Under a humanity and circular economy, you would always have food on your table. This is the main reason Governments and corporations get away with what they do. They set person against person for money and wealth over that of Health.

The Governments of the World must view the coronavirus pandemic as an example of what will befall them if they do not drastically invest and change their policy towards climate change.

While the UK initial Herd policy re coronavirus was misguided and it accepted the death of people over that of the financial economy of the UK. They have shown some compassion and care to help people and business throughout the UK under their £350 Billion package of aid. However, their lack of drive towards halting climate cancer needs to be challenged and radically changed.

We cannot wait, nor can we allow the people in power to continue destroying earth for wealth creation. The people must remove that power. Activism works. We must all stop Governments around the world from putting wealth before the Health of people.

Likewise this will be a tremendous change for the public, especially people who have amassed wealth. But would you rather have wealth and let your children and others die or choose the righteous path?

If our Governments do not act now to stop climate change, then COVID-19 will be a mere ripple in an Ocean to what will occur with climate change. Your children will not have a future.

We should hold Governments and Leaders who do not act now to stop climate damage accountable for their lack of actions.

In past days of the virus, closing Schools was a debatable subject, what about parents, how will they get to work and earn a living? Parents cannot leave their children with elderly grandparents. Will the Government pay their wage? While school children are less likely to die from the virus, they could be unknown carriers of COVID-19.

Problem: Having no lock-down will assist the virus in spreading. So we are back to lock-down a country or not? The UK Government have now realised that their Herd policy was radically flawed and a lock-down should be mandatory, but perhaps a tad too late.

I further believe that all the social, welfare and financial needs of the public should be met. A lock-down would help slow down the number of infections and deaths while they developed a vaccine. **The lock-down will help our planet and atmosphere recover slightly and that alone will help save people's lives.**

In a nutshell, these are unchartered times for COVID-19 and it's at times like this when your Government shows their true colours. Remember a lock-down and social distancing means exactly that, life will not be normal just now. When it comes to social distancing the First Minister of Scotland Nicola Sturgeon said, *"Life shouldn't feel normal right now, so if your life still feels entirely normal, ask yourself if you are doing the right things."* Everyone needs to play their part and restrict the spread of this virus to please stay at home.

False Statistics by the UK Government and other Countries

After the COBRA meeting Scotland's First Minister, Nicola Sturgeon, following on suit to the UK Government's stance on the COVID-19 pandemic said, *"Unless symptoms do not clear up within a few days, or anyone infected is deteriorating, they need not call their GP or NHS24...**there will not be** routine tests on everyone who has coronavirus symptoms, but surveillance will continue."*

How can this be right? How can the UK or any other country get an accurate picture of how many people are carrying the virus if we do not test? This is another sign of the UK's ignorance do anything constructive in case it upsets their "Financial Economy." And to think that other Governments have constantly said the figures being reported from China are far from the truth. Now it seems fit that the UK Government does likewise. We are being led by idiots of a magnitude unreasonable to accept.

On the other flip side, they have reported that there are not enough testing kits. So again, patients being admitted to hospital, health workers and those of essential services should be tested first, don't you think? But that has not been the case.

The crux of all the statistics that you are seeing and hearing about are like an election poll survey. They are not representative of the complete country or world. These statistics are only showing what has occurred so far in the way of a limited testing base.

Therefore, we are back at the same message... stay home, self-isolate when necessary, maintain a social distance, and only go out for medicine, food and exercise. The elderly and the vulnerable should stay at home and away from the general population, while getting help from others that can drop supplies off at their doorstep.

UK Politics worth Noting:

The public must use their vote to vote people into Government based on their manifesto towards human prosperity and not wealth prosperity.

The UK conservative party did not have a public majority in the 2019 general election. 56.4% of the British people voted against Boris Johnson and the Tory party. Three countries voted against the Tories (Scotland, the North of Ireland and wales) Only England voted for the Tories. The Tories do not have a majority, what they have is a majority of seats that have wielded them the power to be in office. This is wrong and certainly does not represent a true majority of the people.

The majority of the British people do not believe in the Tories nor did they want Boris Johnson in power. Therefore the majority of people informed Boris Johnson that they do not want to leave the EU.

The majority of the people are making it crystal clear that the way parliamentary seats are divided up is wrong and against true justice. Three countries voted against the conservatives in the UK 2019 general election, only 1 country voted for the Tories. Therefore, the UK Government had no right to take the UK out of Europe.

It is an injustice how a Government can be formed by a party that 56.4% of the country voted against.

Party politics must be halted. Party politics is not the way ahead for the future of any democratic country.

The world's Economy

"A world where business is motivated primarily by profit – Is no longer an option" Sir Richard Branson

The world's economy and COVID-19, you could say that this virus has not only attacked humans but has also attacked the economies of the world. It has forced Governments to provide financial support to populations at a level never witnessed before.

The world will soon be engulfed in a financial recession of the biggest proportion ever. How the world Governments deal with this will separate the good from the evil. People should come first. It should boil down to one quote, *"Health and personal prosperity should always come first before wealth and financial prosperity."* Quote by Dave Smith.

The simplistic view: There should be no billionaires in this world. That money needs to be taken back and given to the people, after all it was the people who gave them those profits of wealth. Business and Company profits need to be capped. We need smaller businesses and not huge multinational corporations.

The West Australian Government has announced an economic stimulus package worth $607 million to stave off the effects of the coronavirus outbreak. Source ABC.net.au

The Irish Government have developed a new financial support payment to be available to all employees and the self-employed who have lost employment due to a downturn in economic activity caused by the COVID-19 pandemic.

The Department of Employment Affairs and Social Protection [Ireland] are introducing measures to provide income support to people affected by COVID-19.

"3 major changes have been announced:

- *The current 6-day waiting period for Illness Benefit will not* apply to anyone who has COVID-19 or is in medically-required self-isolation

- The personal rate of Illness Benefit will increase from €203 per week to €305 per week for a maximum of 2 weeks medically-required self-isolation or for the full duration of absence from work following a confirmed diagnosis of COVID-19

- The normal social insurance requirements for Illness Benefit will be changed." Source: https://www.gov.ie/

The UK Government has announced the following:

"Those who are not eligible for SSP, for example, the self-employed or people earning below the Lower Earnings Limit of £118 per week, can now more easily make a claim for Universal Credit or Contributory Employment and Support Allowance:

- For the duration of the outbreak, the Universal Credit Minimum Income Floor will be temporarily relaxed...

- people will be able to claim Universal Credit ... without the current requirement to attend a job Centre if they are advised to self-isolate

- contributory Employment and Support Allowance will be payable, at a rate of £73.10 a week if you are over 25, for eligible people affected by COVID-19 or self-isolating in line with advice from Day 1 of sickness, rather than Day 8.

The Government has announced a new £500 million Hardship Fund so Local Authorities can support economically vulnerable people and households..." Source from: gov.uk

What about their mortgage or rent, I hope and assume that it will also be covered? What about peoples other bills? Will the Government force lenders to stop court actions against people who cannot afford to pay? Will the courts allow the coronavirus to be extenuating circumstances?

What will your country offer financially to help people out of hardship, and will it be enough of a financial effort?

With so many business soon to suffer financially, the true colours of our Governments will soon rear their sting, bite or kiss?

The question on every persons mind including the owners and directors of businesses, 'will the Government provide them with funds to remain financially above water?' What about the self-employed, will the Government pay their way?

UPDATE: The UK Government has provided a £350 Billion package to help people and businesses, including mortgage and rent assistance. (19th March 2020) The UK Government have announced that they will pay 80% of the self-employed profits averaged over a three-year period. They have also announced that key workers will receive an increase in wages.

I'm sure that Governments around the world including the UK will continue to provide updates as more ambiguity arises from the COVID-19 virus crisis.

UK Government spending and revenue

Chart 1: Public sector spending 2020-21

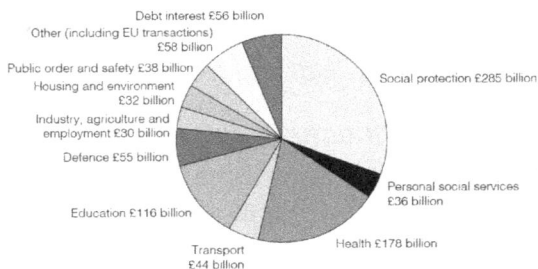

Debt interest £56 billion
Other (including EU transactions) £58 billion
Public order and safety £38 billion
Housing and environment £32 billion
Industry, agriculture and employment £30 billion
Defence £55 billion
Education £116 billion
Transport £44 billion
Social protection £285 billion
Personal social services £36 billion
Health £178 billion

Figures may not sum due to rounding
Illustrative allocations to functions are based on HMT analysis including capital consumption figures from the Office for National Statistics

Source: Office for Budget Responsibility and HM Treasury calculations

Chart 2: Public sector current receipts 2020-21

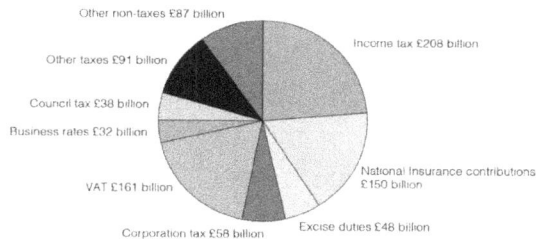

Other non-taxes £87 billion

Other taxes £91 billion

Council tax £38 billion

Business rates £32 billion

VAT £161 billion

Corporation tax £58 billion

Excise duties £48 billion

National Insurance contributions £150 billion

Income tax £208 billion

Figures may not sum due to rounding.
Other taxes includes capital taxes, stamp duties, vehicle excise duties and other smaller tax receipts. Other non-taxes includes interest and dividends, gross operating surplus and other smaller non-tax receipts.

Source: Office for Budget Responsibility and HM Treasury calculations

Extract and source of above charts:
https://www.gov.uk/Government/publications/budget-2020-documents/budget-2020

Because of Lock down and self-isolating for COVID-19 the estimated loss in taxation income using the diagrams above:

- Loss of £8 Billion in Business rates (3 months)

- Loss of £42 Billion in Income Tax (3 months) this also includes a tax adjustment for tax on the 80% of wage. It does not include the 80% wage that the Government have guaranteed to pay.

- Loss of £36 Billion in VAT (3 months)

- Loss of £12 Billion in corporation tax (3 months)

- Loss of £44 Billion in other taxes (3 months)

Additional Expenses to Diagram 1 above:

- £350 Billion announced for aid to offset COVID-19 financial personal and business difficulties.

That is a total estimated loss of £500 Billion for 3 months of lock-down. [Add back Income: Income tax received by people still working e.g. Shop and Businesses and NHS etc.]

I would estimate that the COVID-19 **final bill could even exceed £1 Trillion plus over the next year.** That's assuming that the Government will continue to offer aid and bail out all the business that may face bankruptcy.

What I will guarantee is that they will expect the public to make this shortfall up when 'business as normal' resumes? It could mean higher taxes or additional Government borrowing. However, there could be another way out of this financial depression. I suggest that the world draws a line under all of this additional virus spending and write it off, without getting one penny back from the people. The USA have another way of doing this and they have said they will print more money and loan it to the Federal Reserve while issuing IOU's. There will be no more additional taxes to the people. What will the UK and other countries do? This USA method under current world economic models doesn't stand tall, but then again as Trump as stated many times before America will do what it damn well pleases to do. So buy a USA treasury bond today ☺

As long as any COVID-19 economic recovery post plans do not affect climate change then we should all be ok. If the USA president can print more money for a virus, then it sure as hell can do that to stop climate change to.

Governments and Politician's cannot be allowed to use COVID-19 to avert climate change protests and campaigns. What we could find in the aftermath is crooked Politician's trying to circumvent what is needed to be done to avert our climate emergency. It is possible that such individuals will play on the dire economic times that we will be facing in their attempt to put climate change on the shelf. This cannot be allowed to happen as it will surely seal the fate for our children's future.

We must embrace COVID-19 and thank it for showing us the light, for providing people with the downtime that they needed and for giving us a second chance for life to remain on earth. **To our Politician's and world leaders DO NOT FUCK this opportunity up.**

What is brilliant is the commitment that the UK treasury is putting into helping people through the COVID-19 era. If our Governments did this all of the time, them what a world it would be to live in.

Health before wealth is the best for any situation, and it's the only way forward for a sustainable, green and humanistic future.

The UK Government has announced that it will help renters and those with a mortgage and that any repossession or eviction from properties will stop while this pandemic continues. Consumers who have credit cards, hire purchase, and loans will also be given a break from payments and additional interest, plus their credit reference will not be affected. Check other Government websites for information on your own country.

Until more is known and a vaccine has been developed these times are going to be scary for everyone throughout the world. So please spare a thought for others in other countries that may not have the same level of support that we have within developed countries.

Air quality and the UK admission of liability

"Cleaner vehicles will improve air quality. The Government is committed to bringing roadside concentrations of polluting nitrogen dioxide gas within legal limits in the shortest time. The Budget therefore allocates an added £304 million to enable local authorities to take immediate steps to reduce nitrogen dioxide emissions. This brings the total amount that Government has provided to affected local authorities to £880 million, meeting the Government's obligations to every affected local authorities." Extract from the March 2020 Budget.

"Legal limits," interesting but a word that can be manipulated. What Governments say is legal limits, might not be true legal limits for your absolute safety. Their determination of legal limits will be based on the economic model, in other words wealth generation rather than Health generation.

From the above statement you can clearly see **that the Government is admitting liability for vehicle pollution.** This pollution is responsible for more deaths via cancer, heart and respiratory cancers than COVID-19. Yet we still drive or walk along these polluted roads, we still drive our cars, there is no self-isolating when it comes to air pollution. And you will catch cancer from this pollution.

The mind-set of our Governments is mind boggling, but they are only people like us. How can we self-isolate over COVID-19 and still allow pollution to murder millions? Electric vehicles and green energy needs to be available at affordable prices for everyone.

They must make mandatory Government loans and grants available. Governments could introduce a policy of automatically approving funding for electric vehicles after it makes car manufactures sell cars at affordable prices. The time to nationalise vehicle and energy companies should be a consideration for Governments.

COVID-19 is helping to heal the planet and our health

As a child I remember growing up in my town, there is one particular road on the outskirts that had one road death. Sadly despite many request nothing was done to remove this danger. This stretch on the road was literally a death trap, you did not need a degree to come to that conclusion. Then a second, fifth, and finally 10 deaths occurred before the authorities decided that it was a death trap. Then and only then did they do something about it. 10 People had to sacrifice their life before they did anything to stop any more deaths. The authorities ignored the warning signs until activists stepped in.

Sadly I have witnessed this on many other occasions throughout the world. Why can't Governments and officials act with the speed that is needed to stop life from being lost? Is it a sickness that people in power possess? How many have to die before we do anything concrete and constructive to stop deaths?

The massive lock-down throughout the world has stopped air travel, cars and industry. This has resulted in a huge reduction in pollution and that is saving lives and saving our earth. When we come out at the other end of COVID-19 Governments of the world have to stop climate pollution and fossil fuel use with an urgency of the COVID-19 era.

"Given the huge amount of evidence that breathing dirty air contributes heavily to premature mortality...Burke calculates and states, this has probably saved the lives of 4,000 children under 5 and 73,000 adults over 70 in China. That's significantly more than the current global death toll from the virus itself."

Source:https://www.msn.com/en-gb/news/techandscience/new-evidence-shows-how-covid-19-has-affected-global-air-pollution/ar-BB11jGwt?ocid=spartandhp

One thing for sure is that COVID-19 has helped climate change, by reducing the amount of pollution. The drastic reduction in vehicle use, manufacturing, flights and manufacturing energy has been a fresh breath for our climate and our health. This slight reduction proves that with positive change, people's lives will be saved, and together we can all make an enormous difference.

After COVID-19 if society and the world returns to its normal fossil fuel pollutions then the fate of millions of lives will be in the balance. If the estimate by Burke is accurate, then at the very least millions of lives around the world will be saved. But we don't need Burke or any other scientist to remind us of the deaths by cancer that are caused by pollution. It is clear for all to witness and see in their own families and in the documented statistics of cancer deaths.

If we cannot accept the death of 101,577 people around the world because of COVID-19 (As at 10th April 2020) then how can Governments allow millions of people to die each year from cancer due to pollution? It makes little sense. People who die from cancer should not be collateral damage for fossil fuel companies and other polluters. The Governments and local authorities need to make a stand now and stop these deaths.

The number of COVID-19 reported cases and deaths in China has levelled off. For the last few days it has established to be less than 50 new cases per day. That's three months since the outbreak. The rest of the world are seeing infections increase some at dramatic and concerning rates. However, the accurate picture cannot be determined because there is not enough testing being carried out, so is far from clear. What we also have to be mindful about is that China acted a lot quicker in its lock-down than any other European or world country. Therefore, it is highly possible that infections and deaths could become a lot more around the world than those in China.

Did the lock-downs come too late in the democratic countries of the world? Time will surely tell.

This is a time for the world to come together and

Help each other

"Austerity: It's a campaign of budget cutting that Britain's Conservative-led Government began in 2010 in the aftermath of the global financial panic of 2008, the most crippling economic downturn since the Great Depression."

Countries are totally at the mercy of financial services and a financial economy. The endeavour for wealth, power and fame is what drove Donald Trump and many other billionaires towards their goals. The world's economy has suffered some severe recessions since the Second World War but then came the slump of 2008/09. That was declared the worst of all, at least until COVID-19 arrived.

COVID-19 will beat all financial depressions throughout the world hands down. But it need not do so, the world has a fresh opportunity to change its financial model towards that of a humanitarian model and solution, one where the world joins together and works as a unified team.

A time when all prejudices are set aside, a time when the universe can witness humans come together for all species and biodiversity on earth.

It will take bold leadership from the Governments of the world, but this could be out last chance at saving earth from a future of extinction.

This is a time for the world to come together and help each other. I have heard of retired health workers and other essential service workers offering their help if needed. In these uncertain times we don't know who will be unable to work due to infection, however it is great that people are putting themselves forward as standbys to ensure that essential services still continue.

Religion

It's sad when the rest of the world is constructively doing something in their attempts at halting the spread of COVID-19. Then you read about some religions counter acting everyone's hard work at social distancing, self-isolating and locking down, all done in the name of a person's faith and religion.

"The day after Pope Francis delivered a blessing in an empty St Peter's Square, watched on television by about 11 million people, Sunday services were held at some of Russia's largest religious sites after Orthodox Church leaders said they expressed religious freedom." Report by The Guardian newspaper. And likewise as I reported the Jewish Funeral in Brooklyn, USA.

How idiotic and self-centred can a religion be? With a deadly virus, it does not entitle religion to any such expression of freedom by manipulating others to become infected. That religion will follow the same rules as every other person in this world. Full stop!

Only a person not of sane mind or with no due care of other people in the world would recommend its followers to forgo social distancing over a church congregation, funeral or Rabbi Funeral meeting.

Matthew 6:5 "And when you pray, you must not be like the hypocrites. For they love to stand and pray in the synagogues and at the street corners, that they may be seen by others."

Are they hypocrites or do they not give a fuck for other human life?

Ghost Town's & Humour

Towns and city centres became ghost towns, few people milling around. People prefer to stay at home and not become infected. Cafes, restaurants, bars, non-essential shops and supermarkets have all closed their doors. As from 24th March 2020 all non-essential UK shops have been ordered to close their door. Childminders have been told that only children of essential workers can be cared for.

On the funny side, I have seen and heard many humorous takes on the coronavirus. *"A priest made a statement that the person who stole the churches toilet roll will suffer in hell when the devil sticks a red hot poker up his arse."* We need humour to keep us all sane.

Scan QR image below to watch a Funny video explaining the Coronavirus by John Oliver. **Warning: Do not drink bleach, it will kill you.**

https://qrs.ly/1hbddm6

They announced that Boris Johnson the UK prime minister has joined some other world leaders and celebrities that have been tested positive for the Novel Coronavirus, COVID-19. This shows that no one is invincible from the virus. But on a humorous note, the picture on the next page was tweeted to me. To the unknown photographer and creator of this, well done. But alas Boris's work contract will ensure that he does not get SSP or 80% pay...but full pay, so thumbs up Mr Johnson.

Emotional Wellbeing during the COVID-19 Outbreak

On a more serious note, keep an eye on your young children and teenagers. It has been reported that isolation and a change in normal social activities have created a lot of anxiety and depression for many people. Some have gone as far as suicide.

Please help your children and teenagers through this life-changing event. You are the adults, now live up to this challenge. Take precautions seriously but no not induce fear onto your children. Explain and give them the facts without the stampede of concern. Do not turn to alcohol or drugs to ease through these difficult times, doing so will only make your situation far worse.

Coping Tips, people that are feeling emotional distress related to COVID-19 can take actions to help support themselves and others. Scan to go to the suicide prevention website on COVID-19.

https://qrs.ly/axbe0uu

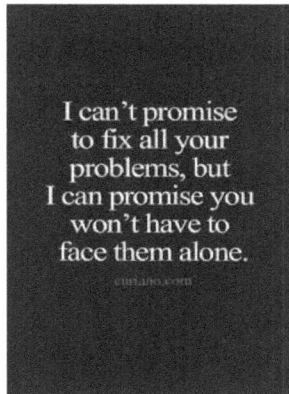

I can't promise to fix all your problems, but I can promise you won't have to face them alone.

Be there for your child, teenager, family and others. These are trying times for everyone.

Short animation for young children to help them better understand COVID-19

https://qrs.ly/kwbe0ui

Answering Kids questions on Coronavirus

https://qrs.ly/8cbe0uh

This webinar offers clinical guidance on the newly emerged Coronavirus strain (COVID-19) and strategies for paediatricians

https://qrs.ly/albe0ur

Dirty Money

Before the lock-down, I went to the post office and bank. The tellers had plastic gloves on their hands. I witnessed several tellers handle money then immediately touch their mouth and face with the same gloved hands. It's a habit of ritual, difficult to stop when you probably have being doing the same for years.

I asked one teller why the gloves? She replied we are dealing with "Dirty Money," I told her that she has always been dealing with dirty money, what's the difference now? I don't want to catch the COVID-19 virus, she replied. I asked her, "Where you never scared about catching the flu virus from this dirty money before?" More people have died from the flu virus, or cancer via pollution than what the statistics display regarding coronavirus (at present, but those figures could change, however millions would need to die each year to exceed the deaths per year from cancer).

But people are genuinely scared about coronavirus, this is a virus that will change people's daily life. It is a virus that can kill those more vulnerable and now even some healthy young people are dying from the virus. It will change the financial economies of the world. I also hope that it will change the viewpoint of the public and Governments on what needs to be done with immediate effect towards eliminating climate cancer.

I watched a Netflix documentary called 'Dirty Money.' But before I talk about that, I want to tell you this short story... When I was a child my Mum and Dad told me, "If you want to find out how clean a restaurant is, visit their toilet first before ordering food. If it's clean, there is a far better chance that the staff are meeting hygiene and business standards, so it should be an enjoyable experience to dine there."

The moral of my story is keep your business clean and people will respect you and will look forward to dealing with you. Now back to the Dirty Money documentary, after watching a few episodes, I was in moral disgust, I cried for the people who were forced to suffer and became despaired at how the rich can abuse others all in the name of money and wealth accumulation and have the force of justice behind them, and it is scandalous. Law is forced upon us therefore they should provide each person with the same legal defence. They should never allow the rich to circumvent law because they can afford a better legal team. That is not true justice, nor is it a law that we can allow to continue any longer.

a)...The president of the USA and his son-in-law adviser is far from clean. Jared Corey Kushner has a property business and uses scumbag tactics to make money from the tenants while they live in squalor. The fact that he is a senior adviser to a president is a disgrace, he believes, like Trump, that he can get away with what he does while silently giving a middle finger to the American people. He and Trump have made disgusting amounts of wealth from the backs of all the little people. And when they get into financial trouble, it's the Government and the little people who bail them out so that they can become billionaires yet again. This has to stop!

b)...The USA Government backed up with corrupt solicitors, judges and a legal system that creates financial and mental hardships for the elderly through forced Guardianships. Please watch this Dirty money Netflix episode, and if you don't feel any moral disgust, then you need to take a good look at yourself in the mirror.

c)...Formosa the plastics manufacturer polluted land, ocean and humans through their lack of concern for their employees, and the people living in the vicinity. They destroyed the environment for profit & wealth before the health of people and planet.

USA Government officials and leaders have been paid off with party donations and employment for locals while American workers and the environment suffered.

In a, b and c above their houses are far from clean. They need to be closed down. Get rid of Trump and his administration. VOTE FOR A CLIMATE FIRST PRESIDENT, instead of people with nothing really to offer a country apart from, "Look at me did I not do well, I've made billions of dollars at the expense of the little people."

Dirty money is why very little has been done about curbing the climate change disaster. That would mean closing all oil, coal, gas, plastic and other polluting companies. These companies have a vested interest in the policy making of your Governments. Trump loves them, he believes that the sun shines out of their arses, and Trump thinks climate change is nonsense. He and his administration are investing our future in additional fossil fuel production. What Trump loves is money and the power over the little people. Trump also thought he knew everything about Coronavirus, did he not? After all his genetics from his scientist uncle infected him with COVID-19 knowledge.

In a nutshell, please watch that documentary, and if after watching you feel no disgust and hatred towards these scumbags, then you are a lost soul and are here on earth purely for the money and wealth.

True humanity is Health and People Prosperity over wealth and financial prosperity.

You have been given an opportunity to breathe earth's air, don't fuck it up anymore. The time for health and human prosperity has arrived.

Coronavirus is the light from the universe, you have been given a second chance to mend your ways. Do the right thing, stop pollution and stop fossil fuel use.

Death Statistics

China Death Statistics:

COVID-19 deaths at 16/3/20: 3,213
Road accident deaths in 2016: 290,000
Cancer deaths: 7,500 per day
Number of people aged of 65 and over: 123 million

Source:https://www.abc.net.au/news/2016-03-24/chinas-cancer-rates-exploding-study-says/7272266

UK Death Statistics

COVID-19 deaths at 23/3/20: 335
Road deaths in 2018: 1,710 seriously injured and deaths 26,610
Cancer deaths: 165,000 per year
Number of people aged of 65 and over: 11.98 million

Source: https://www.gov.uk/ and https://www.cancerresearchuk.org/

USA Death Statistics

COVID-19 deaths at 23/3/20: 517
Road deaths in 2018: 33,654
Cancer deaths: 609,640 per year
Number of people aged of 65 and over: 49.2 million

Source: https://www.cancer.gov/

Italy Death Statistics

COVID-19 deaths at 16/3/20: 6,077
Road deaths in 2018: 3,325
Cancer deaths (2014): 177,301 per year
Number of people aged of 65 and over: 13.6 million

Source: https://www.itf-oecd.org/ and https://www.ncbi.nlm.nih.gov/pmc/articles/PMC6406941/

The table above was created by the author from data from the above sources.

From the country statistics above you can clearly see the numbers of people being killed via vehicles and cancer pollution are extremely high. Yet, we have never went into lock-down over those deaths. It's business as usual.

So what does business as usual tell you? How come people are more scared of coronavirus which has fewer deaths as compared to the cancer statistic's above?

COVID-19 has the power and speed to infect every person on earth as it is transmitted from person to person, and that's a potential recipe for millions to die via COVID-19. Therefore, a lock-down is essential to stop the spread of COVID-19. Cancer is not caught from person to person. However, cancer can be caught form the air we breathe, and if a person is vulnerable then they have a greater chance of contracting respiratory or cancer illnesses via the air we breathe.

After coronavirus slows down, will people become more aware of cancer deaths and stop the use of fossil fuel products and pollution? Time will surly tell.

One of the major differences between COVID-19 and cancer deaths is that people don't have to stop using their cars or change their polluting ways because to do that would be a major upheaval for them. COVID-19 is a temporary setback until a vaccine is found, then its business as usual. With possible higher taxes to come to pay for the downturn in the coronavirus affected economy.

If COVID-19 joined forces with the other statistic's and murdered people at the same rate as cancer would people still be in lock-down or would it just be accepted as another way to die for the vulnerable and elderly? Will that then become the acceptable norm of deaths as has human cancer become?

The sad reality is people will not ditch their car or dirty business or holiday flights to stop co2 pollution. Michael O'Leary Ryanair's CEO's made that clear when he stated that *"they should shoot all environmentalists."* Did he go to jail for that comment? No! But hey, if you stood on one of his Boeing 737 aircraft and said jokingly there's a bomb on here, would you be let off? Don't think so, you would be in jail. That's legal and inconsistent justice.

Yet Governments will still let over 600,000 people in the USA die from cancer. You can remedy cancer by stopping fossil fuels and pollution production. The number of cases of cancer each year is rising dramatically, yet we fanny around and let these large corporations murder us.

Human and Climate Cancer

"Human Cancer is Climate Cancer. They are both the same. They are both intrinsically connected." **Dave Smith.**

The word cancer sends chills throughout your body and fear sets in when a doctor informs you that you have cancer. For many people they have had suspicions but did nothing about it, they were in denial. Then at the last moment they clamber for help, to get support and possible an operation, but for the majority it's too late. For some people they never knew they had it until it was too late.

The above statement is also true for our climate change problem. For some they are in denial, for some it is through greed that they don't want any change. For others they believe that our Governments are taking proper care of the situation, but they are not.

In reality if our Governments don't act quicker and halt fossil fuel use and pollution then climate cancer will murder your children's future.

You don't want that to happen, do you?

Contagion

- Globally, it is estimated that there were 18.1 million fresh cancer cases and 9.6 million cancer deaths in 2018

- The Global Flu outbreak in 1918 killed 50 million people.

- The Spanish flu killed more people than World War One.

So with all that it mind, yes it is right to take every precaution that we can with COVID-19.

It is a virus that we don't know enough about and there are no developed vaccines as yet. People don't want to die, right?

The primary difference about COVID-19 vs the flu. The flu is a seasonal virus, and we are all used to it, plus there are flu vaccines available. But still millions die from the flu.

Whereas COVID-19 is an unknown virus, could it be seasonal or all year round? The fact that over one million people have become infected is proof that it isn't going anywhere else in a hurry. It will remain and take its place in the arena of diseases that infect and sometimes kill the human population. Therefore, a vaccine is highly desirable. Recent reports is now suggesting that the Novel Coronavirus COVID-19 could become a seasonal event similar to the flu. Will countries continue their lock-down year after year? Or will COVID-19 cases and deaths become accepted into society as was the flu and cancer, and life will continue with no lock-downs or interventions until something new rears its ugly head? I guess time will only tell.

What is the difference between COVID-19 and Climate Cancer? Both can kill people, both can be cured. Both require drastic changes in our current way of life. But to date only COVID-19 has had any proper Government action taken with an immediate urgency and action plan to halt the spread. Climate Cancer is killing you Governments need to do more to halt climate change.

However, what we all should have an issue with is: We are facing a pathway to an unchangeable extinction level event within the next 10 to 40 years via climate change. Yet our Governments, leaders and Politician's throughout the world are dragging their feet, and making slow progress. No major reductions to fossil fuel emissions throughout the world. In fact it's still rising and some countries are increasing their production of fossil fuels including the USA. The Climate Emergency will create a far larger problem than COVID-19 will ever create.

At first I thought the almost immediate Government action [took 2 to 3 months for action re COVID-19 for some countries] was because of the coronavirus emergency being right now. But the climate emergency is happening right now is it not?

No, I mean coronavirus is effecting people right now, people are dying from COVID-19, and people are being infected by it right now! But so is Climate pollution, people are being murdered by cancer, heart disease and respiratory illnesses directly because of climate pollution from fossil fuel and tobacco manufactures to name a few, this is happening every single day, just like COVID-19 only climate cancer is killing millions of people each year.

We have thousands of deaths every single day throughout the world because of lung cancer, heart illness, and respiratory illness because of climate pollutions.

Yet more is being done to stop the spread of COVID-19 than the spread of an extinction level event (climate change.) The COVID-19 virus is not an extinction level event, yet it is getting more support from countries for action than what climate change has every got. Now that is sick and extremely worrying.

Be more afraid of climate change and pollution than COVID-19. COVID-19 is a pandemic, climate change and pollution is a murderous horrific horror event that will eventually make COVID-19 look like a kindergarten party.

Governments are acting immediately to try and stop COVID-19. But our climate emergency has been last on their list, even despite

Governments declaring a climate emergency. Their words are frivolous, its immediate action that is required and not just words.

Governments listened to health Organisation's, scientists and advisors and then declared a Coronavirus pandemic. Within weeks parts of China locked down. Two months later the entire country of Italy locked down, almost three months later the UK was locked down and with many other countries restricting travel unless warranted.

165,000 people in the UK die with cancer every year. 609,000 die from cancer each year in the USA. Most of this cancer if not all directly results from burning fossil fuels, plastics pollution, tobacco smoking and second hand smoke and unhealthy life choices. Yet our Governments have not acted with the same contingency, action plan or gumption for the climate emergency as they have done for the coronavirus.

Donald Trump, believes he knows it all, after all he declared himself all knowledgeable about coronavirus. His acceptance of donations from oil and tobacco companies has insured that the American people will continue to suffer from human cancer, and climate cancer. Trump is a staunch patriot, and he makes sure that you even pay for your own health treatment for both cancers that he allows to continue, all done through greed and wealth accumulation concepts. Keeping the oil and tobacco companies in business is his prime concern, people's health is not.

In October 2019 they undertook a USA pandemic scenario
"Event 201 was a 3.5-hour pandemic table top exercise that simulated a series of dramatic scenarios, scan QR image below for more details. **2 Months later the genuine thing began.**

Even more interesting, the film "Contagion" premiered on 3rd September 2011 and is horrifically similar to the current COVID-19 pandemic. Well worth a second watch. You will be shocked at how daunting and similar it is to our current COVID-19 pandemic.

EVENT 201 - https://qrs.ly/y4bdvlc

The Movie Contagion, 2011	China	Donald Trump IDIOT-1
Bat Dropped a bit of Banana	Unknown Cause	Trumps uncle passed his science genetics to Trump
Pig eats this piece of Banana	Possibly a Bat borne virus?	So Trumps knows it all.
Pig Slaughtered by Chef	Live animals being slaughtered next to live animals for sale or Lab experiments on bats?	Possibly a Bat borne virus?
Chef shake hands with Beth prior to washing his hands	Possible the same type of transmission	Trump shakes hands with Boris Johnson
Beth first person Infected	Unknown as yet	I'm sure he would take a guess
Infected people travel while infecting others	Infected people travel while infecting others	It's only one person from China, we have it under control
Novel Virus MEV-1	COVID-19	Renames it to "Chinese Virus"
Forsythia	~~No vaccine as yet as per CDC and WHO~~ **December 2020 Vaccine is in use**	**Trumps States it is Chloroquine?**

Why the lack of action for climate cancer?

As I already explained, at first it might appear that it is because coronavirus is spreading as I write. But then so is human cancer, so is the destruction of our planet and environment, (both due to fossil fuel pollution) these two cancers are spreading *"like your house is on fire."* Only the 'people' can put that fire out, Governments won't take the lead in telling fossil fuel companies to 'fuck off our people come first,' we need to do that with activism and to stop buying their products.

We need to force Governments to become more humanistic and develop an economic model suitable for everyone and not just the rich.

Our Governments are being patriotic idiots, they are putting money and financial wealth above your health and that is the totality for their lack of action.

After all, we have been allowing millions of people to die with cancer every year due to fossil fuel pollution. But yes you can get from A to B quicker by car, plane etc. and so forth, you get the picture, right? But yet you do nothing about stopping this madness.

You would rather self-isolate and stockpile foods due to coronavirus than fight a system that is currently and has been for many years murdering your family, friends, children, mother, father, brother, sister and now soon it will be our Earth.

Try living with that! The financial economy does not work for the majority of people. It only works for a few million out of 7.8 Billion people. The rest of the population are the worker ants, who make the wealth and prosperity for those few million. It's time to tell those queen bees enough is enough.

Governments are allowing fossil fuel and tobacco companies to pollute our environment which in turn murders the human population and Earth. All done in the name of wealth and prosperity. It's a false reality, a reality that we need to stop now. It's a false economy and one that needs changed to become a humanitarian one, people need to come first.

Coronavirus has highlighted the need for change. If Governments are taking these precautions over COVID-19 then they surly need to accept that murdering via cancers from fossil fuel pollution, has to be halted.

Our Governments can no longer ignore the World Health Organisation (WHO), the IPCC and the scientific community on climate damage and its pathway to our extinction. You would think If our Governments listened to scientists and the WHO over coronavirus then they must surely now accept their word on climate damage? After all, we see the effects of climate damage and pollution every single day and millions are dying from it each year.

China is experiencing an exploding lung cancer growth, this is directly because of the increase of Chinese work environments and pollution. You have to remember that china's pollution is a direct result of developed countries need for goods to be manufactured and then sent back to USA, UK and Europe. As demand grew for these products so did china's need for more factories and transportation, this required more fuel and energy. The pollution in China has grown exponential based on demand for products to be exported to developed countries (USA, Europe, UK etc.)

The drive for a financial economy at all costs will be the destruction of humanity. Now is the time to act. If complete countries are willing to go into lock down over a killer virus that could have a high recovery rate then they must do likewise to save humanity from climate destruction and extinction that has a low survival rate.

Scan for Coronavirus details and research

World Health Organisation Coronavirus overview

https://qrs.ly/habcxyp

WHO Coronavirus video and questions

https://qrs.ly/hubcxym

Rolling Update on COVID-19

Scan QR code below to be kept up to date with latest COVID-19 Information from the World Health Organisation. (WHO)

https://qrs.ly/z3bcxyd

Scan the QR image below to get a complete MSN search and update of COVID-19 including advice and links to other official bodies.

https://qrs.ly/babduah

Scan the QR below to be kept up to date with WHO situation reports.

https://qrs.ly/lwbcxya

John Hopkins CORONAVIRUS RESOURCE CENTRE

"This website is a resource to help advance the understanding of the virus, inform the public, and brief policymakers to guide a response, improve care, and save lives."

https://qrs.ly/f4bdvkh

Social Distancing

Businesses and shops are putting social distancing measures in place as you can see from the photos below. I particular like the photo I took from our local petrol/food station. They have put in place measures to protect staff from coughs and breathing from the public, by erecting see through barriers between staff and public. As you can see from the photograph, these barriers are sensitive and still allow social interaction and are not by any means offensively placed or a security barrier, well done. It is great to see business adapting to meet the needs of their customers on their own without Government intervention

From the picture below you can see that I purchased a coffee (I had given coffee and tea up, but I indulge in one every month), a bun (unhealthy) and a packet of almonds (healthy). What is sad, all of my purchased items are in throw away packaging (the coffee cup is recyclable.) But I'm annoyed at myself for doing this. I could have brought my own reusable container for the coffee. But during COVID-19 times, the bun has to be wrapped in a plastic wrapper to stop any chance of infection. The almonds I guess I could purchase in bulk without individual wrapping? What about inventing sustainable packaging?

What you can take from my 3 items purchased, is that I'm like most other people out there in the world, we want to do the best for our climate, pollution and waste, etc. But we need help and direction from those in authorities. We need better innovation and creation of sustainable goods, products and packaging. We need to recycle more and buy less crap that we don't need in our lives.

What I know is that I and everyone else needs to change our way of life dramatically. We cannot stand by and assume our Politian's and Governments know better. We need to give them a helping hand to make decisive decisions that will benefit our planet and future life on earth for all generations to come.

Next time you are out shopping take a closer look at the amount of packaging that there is. Most of which comes from plastics. Plastics are bad for pollution and our environment. We need sustainable packing sooner rather than later.

Perhaps businesses can take the lead and make their shops plastic free and have products with no packaging. But what about crisps and many other quick small snacks, as shown above in the photograph? As you can see we need manufacturing and food production to package sustainable or stop producing all the crap that is bad for your health anyway.

Facts, Questions, Reporting, Stats and Climate Justice.

I have picked some random countries to look at questions and reporting, to make you aware of what all countries throughout the world should be doing or asking themselves. How can we make this dire situation better?

Statistics for the North of Ireland

The following statistics are based on the North of Ireland. I would suggest that you research your own local areas wherever you live in the world. Get your information from reliable sources and not fake news sites.

Isolation is the best way to solve COVID-19 until more is known about the virus.

NI Stats as at 11th April 2020:

- **11,765** people have been tested

- **1,717** people have tested positive

- **107** people have died from COVID-19

- **1.882** million is the population of NI

14.6% of people tested are declared positive (1,717)

6.23% of those people declared positive have died. (107 deaths)

0.00625% of the NI population have been tested so far.

As you can see from the limited statistics above isolation can work and the more that people don't abide by the rules then they are the ones responsible for infecting and Killing others.

IRELAND

"On the 10th of April 2020: they confirmed 25 deaths and 480 new cases

The Health Protection Surveillance Centre has today been informed that 25 people diagnosed with COVID-19 in Ireland have died.

Of the 25 deaths:

The median age was 82

The people included 11 females and 14 males

16 of the 28 had an underlying condition

480 new cases of COVID-19 in Ireland have been confirmed. There are now 7054 confirmed cases of COVID-19 in Ireland.

Including test results which have been sent to Germany for testing (which may include tests from older cases) the total figure of those who have been diagnosed with COVID-19 in Ireland now stands at 8,089.

Source: https://www.gov.ie/en/news/7e0924-latest-updates-on-covid-19-coronavirus/#april-10

Could it be that the elderly's immune system is not strong enough regardless of them have underlying health conditions or not? As a matter of urgency the medical research teams need to determine why people with no underlying health conditions are dying regardless of their age. We need to know why? Why are most of the young immune to deaths? These are questions that we need answer for. It is important that these facts are uncovered as soon as possible. If the virus changes its potency, then these questions I have asked will become even more prevalent to safeguard every person.

FRANCE

On the 2nd of April, France announced that they would include deaths from nursing homes in their COVID-19 figures. What about deaths that happened before have these now been included as well? It is stupid to be excluding any deaths from COVID-19 statistical reporting.

We need the verifiable facts from every country in the world, no hiding facts. We should hold any country that hides statistics accountable and responsible.

MEXICO

On the 10th of April Mexico's Ministry of Health reported 3,844 confirmed patients and 233 deaths and that 33,893 had been tested.

The alarming situation about the number of cases and deaths being reported throughout the world is: They are only being declared from people actual tested or from those that have died. The statistics we are getting are not necessarily reflective of the entire population. Testing needs to be rolled out on a wider scale and faster than what is occurring at present.

USA

At 9th April 2020	
The State of New York	
Total number of people Tested	417,885
Total tested Positive	170,512
USA population	330,573,517

The above data was sourced from:
https://covid19tracker.health.ny.gov/

Of the above that tested positive: 45.2% were female, 54.2% were male and 0.6% unknown

The statistics above show that out of the 417,885 people tested, **40%** of those tested in the state of New York are found to **have tested positive**. Now that is quite an alarming result.

If you look at my example on the Brooklyn funeral and how their religion believes that they can mass mourn in close proximity, highlights and demonstrates how this virus is spreading.

USA as at 11th April 2020

- **30%** of the worlds reported cases of COVID-19 infection is within the USA.
- **20%** of USA citizens tested, have tested positive for COVID-19
- **3.7%** of those that are tested positive Die.
- **0.0077%** of the USA population has been tested for COVID-19 as at 11th April 2020.

[World cases 1,700,951 USA cases 503,177]
[In USA 2,538,888 people were tested, 503,177 people were positive with COVID-19]

This would show that despite what Trump originally stated, the USA were pretty well infected from day one. Trumps policy of 'Business as Usual' during the announcement of Coronavirus by the World Health Organisation is directly responsible for the huge number of cases within America? The USA had its first COVID-19 case on 21st January 2020, yet Trump did very little until the middle of March.

Is the USA alone in this? Of course they are not, many countries in the world have been lackadaisical on their testing or have they? What we have to remember is that COVID-19 is new, it takes time to develop reliable kits and get them mobilised for mass population testing.

However, if we take the percentages outlined above then if all the USA was tested then there could be 66 million to 133 million people in the USA infected with COVID-19. That could equate to 2.4 million and upwards in deaths from America alone. These figures are speculative in so far as if the current trend continues that could be the scenario. This could vary dramatically (down or up) based on self-isolation techniques, social distancing and how much of the virus penetrated the public before any lock-down became affective?

The above statistics are based on a current trend and applied to a future that is still yet to arrive. Therefore, while these stats are future trends, the future can be changed. This has already has been demonstrated in China. China's quick response and their country wide lock-down ensured that COVID-19 was kept at a low level. We can see this in the number of cases and deaths within China. As at 11th April 2020, the number of cases in China stands at 81,953 and 3,339 deaths.

So how do we change the future? Quite simply by following the same set of rules as did China. Same set of rules that Italy, UK, France and other countries are now putting in place. This means that we need a larger lock-down on people's movements, while putting in place an infrastructure that will keep the population in food and health. Everything else should be secondary.

The lack of speed to which countries reacted to COVID-19 after the WHO announcement is abysmal. However, that is now in the past, the future can be bright if we all follow the same rules and that includes everyone even people of religious faiths. The rules apply to everyone, there should be no special exceptions.

What I will say is that the USA president Donald Trump was totally complacent on the original news of the outbreak, he believed that he knew it all and that it would not reach American soil. And then when it did, what did that scoundrel of a president do? He blamed the Chinese by renaming COVID-19 to become the "Chinese Virus" Oh merciful God, how could and how can the people of American allow an IDIOT-1 billionaire of a person become and remain the president of America? Or perhaps later we discover that Trump was only acting on advice from his advisors, the whole lot of them should be scrapped.

Retesting

We need those that have been tested positive to be retested at later stages to see if the virus can re-infect a person or have the infected gained some sort of immunity from their first infection. The unwelcome news if a person can be re-infected then it will be much harder to stop this virus and a vaccine would be the only alternative to mass deaths.

The Vaccine

Those that are not becoming infected or are becoming infected but have no major symptoms. I believe that they may hold the key for a vaccine. A research team needs commissioned to investigate this further.

Climate Justice

If the world's Governments can do this vast mobilisation and disregard to the financial economy over COVID-19, then they also need to be doing the same effort for a bigger pandemic soon to hit earth. And that's Climate Cancer, sadly for me I won't be alive** when the true effect of climate change affects earth and its populations. By then I will have died and moved onto my next journey in 'life and self.' But my children and their children will be bang right in the middle of this known and well documented pandemic. And with COVID-19 the future can be changed, but only if we act now and soon enough without waiting to the very last minute. And before I die, I must maintain a campaign for climate justice and so should you.

** If you believe in reincarnation, then it is vitally important that you do something major to stop climate cancer, because you will be reborn into this madness of a climate pandemic of extinction proportions. If you do not believe in reincarnation, then do you think for one second that any god would welcome you in to heaven with open arms when you have fucked the planet and the people that he gave to you? And please don't think you can confess your sins before you die and that you're out of the shit. That won't cut it either, so think again for those that believe they can do what they want because of a confessional scam.

The fight for climate justice includes fighting corporate globalisation, these industries are the ones being supported by Governments, and these are the industries that are destroying earth and your children's future so that they can get richer. Wealth over Health will be the destruction of humankind. Therefore, if you don't do something now about climate change, then you are totally fucked regardless of your spiritual or religious belief.

Posting Blame on China

Now fingers are being pointed at China, in particular by the USA, remembering that their initially handling of the Coronavirus was negligent in its totality. They had a president saying, "It might get a wee bit bigger or it might not." Trump handled this pandemic in the way he handles all matters of necessity that does not fit with his personal wealth agenda. Trump, is a denier who enlists the support of deceitful and lying aids… "It's freezing here, give us some global warming….I'm cancelling billions of dollars for climate change…"

Now he wants to point a finger and blame China. Trump accepts no responsibility for anything. China had nothing to win by allowing a virus to infect people globally. After all the virus kills mostly the elderly and vulnerable and not people who could go to war against a nation.

Moreover, purposely infecting the world affects China's economy. And as we can see in the news Trumps war against China and the trade between these two countries is sickening. Trump chastised Boris Johnson the UK prime minister for allowing Huawei (Chinese Telecommunication Company) to be accepted for a UK contract. Just a reminder to Trump and his administration you do not own the rest of the world, OK!

The Americans are great for their conspiracy theories and so are many others throughout the world. In reality conspiracy theories distracts people from the real agendas and hence fixing the problems sooner rather than later or never and is an attempt to pass the blame onto others.

Now the Americans state that they will hold those responsible accountable, that's a statement that could induce a world war. They suggest that it was a cover up by the Chinese. Their exact words are "U.S. Intelligence Officials Believe China Covered up the Severity..." The key word is "Believe," it's not an actual fact but a mere possibility. This same US intelligence office were also making claims and beliefs against their own US president Donald Trump [Russian election meddling and more...]

Now really who and what can you believe when it comes from the mouths of an administration that is hell bend in denying and twisting the facts, both in relation to the coronavirus and climate change to name only a few?

Misinformation and slowness of information from China is what many countries now believe to be the case. But if it was done on purpose, then this is still yet to be proved to be within a shadow of doubt. But in reality China had nothing to gain from maliciously releasing such a virus. What would be more understating is that it could have been a mistake or error of some sort? Another point to remember is that all countries knew of China's impending lock down, yet other European countries and the USA did not lockdown until 2 to over 3 months later. If they had acted at the same time as China then they would have saved many thousands of lives. That is true and a fact and not a "belief."

China until we know otherwise with undeniable facts is only guilty of a lack of freedom. People have a birth right to freedom, pure equality and a life of freedom from pain, misery, poverty and homelessness.

Some activities to keep you and

Your little ones busy and amused at home

Here are some items you can do, make your own list and enhance on the basic details below. These are just to get your creative juices flowing.

1. Have a wheelbarrow race

2. Lay on the ground and slither like a snake.

3. Have a pillow fight.

4. Play catch with a stuffed animal.

5. Roll up a pair of socks and see who can throw them into a bucket, keep track of the scores

6. Go around the house and get the children to wipe the counters and surfaces with a bacterial wipe.

7. Play water balloon catch, best done in your garden.

8. Spin in a circle but be careful of objects around you. Don't do this too often as it can cause dizziness.

9. Pull your child around on a sheet or blanket.

10. Plant or repot plants or create your own herb garden.

11. Dare, lick lemons, make sure each person has their own personal piece of lemon to lick.

12. Play floor or table football by blowing a cotton ball across a table. You score if you blow it off the other person's end.

13. Play a listening game. Sit quietly and guess the sounds you hear.

14. Play catch with a balloon

15. Trace your hands on a piece of paper and colour it in

16. Using a blindfold, take turns in guessing different smells, e.g. water, milk, apples oranges etc.

17. Bake some cookies

18. Make pancakes

19. Cook lunch and dinner, everyone has a task from peeling potatoes to washing dishes.

20. Hours of fun making slime, go to this video to see how's it's done:

https://qrs.ly/g6bdo0q

21. Do some homework, parents have to try what the child has to do. Good luck on that task!

22. Help your child with some homework

23. Let your child help with some housework, cleaning tables, floor, counters, etc.

24. Make up a song or story together. Get the Story Lyrics book.

25. Play I-Spy with my little eye, something beginning with B

26. Sing and do, Head shoulders knees and toes, knees and toes, eyes and mouth, ears and nose.

27. Play "do what I tell you and not what I do" Touch your toes, touch your elbow. Then see who wins the game. So you say touch your toes but you physically touch your head. Those that touch their head are out of that game. Practice first.

28. Let the kids raid your closet and put on a fashion show.

29. Read books together.

30. Get a deck of cards and teach or play some card games.

31. Learn how to play backgammon

32. Watch a film together as a family, make some popcorn and drinks.

33. Write a letter instead of using text messages

34. Make some chocolate rice crispy cakes. You will need rice crispy or cornflakes, and some cooking chocolate. Melt the chocolate and mix in the rice crispy then let them set in a baking tray. Cut into squares when cooled down.

35. Play some indoor keep fit exercises.

36. Play with dominoes or snakes and ladders

37. Play noughts and crosses. Get this book

https://qrs.ly/zhbdo5e

38. Make paper-bag puppets and put on a show.

39. Make a bird feeder for the garden

40. Learn to do something new, like computer programming, cooking. There are lots of YouTube videos to learn from.

41. Do a jigsaw

42. Build a model ship, aircraft, car etc.

43. Make your own guess who I'm game. Stick a name of a person on each other's head and each person has to guess who it is by giving a clue.

44. Have a karaoke night.

45. Play musical chairs

46. Play musical statue, last person to stop dancing or moving when music stops is out, keep going until the last person wins.

47. Make your own set of home bowling, using plastic cartons and roll up socks to make a ball.

48. Make an indoor obstacle course

49. Get some activity books.

50. Pillow fight

51. Make a sand painting, get a board map out the drawing by marker, and then put glue on small parts at a time while you add sand to it. Use colouring to change colour of sand.

52. Everyone sleeps downstairs with torches as their light.

53. Bottle flip competition.

54. Search online for science experiments that you can safely learn at home.

55. Stain Glass window: Tape a piece of plastic to the window. Cut out shapes from coloured paper. And stick these shapes to the plastic taped on the window.

56. Racing ping balls along a course that you have taped to the floor. Cut out cardboard and lay it on the floor making a racing course with two lanes. Then you blow a cotton or ping ball along the course to see who wins. Or you could use a round sweet but DON'T eat it afterwards.

57. Target golf. Get a cardboard box. Cut out small doors along one side. Each person has to roll a ping-pong ball or something round into the doors. Each door has a different value the person with the highest score after 4 throws wins.

58. Play darts

59. Make an indoor climbing frame. This is a project that could take a few days to make.

60. Cave drawing: Sit inside a cardboard box and colour in or draw on the insides.

61. Large size tic-tac-toe. Get paper plates and paint x and o on them. Then put tape off the floor to make your x and o table.

62. Balloon painting, Blow up the balloon then dip it into paint and then stamp your sheet of paper.

63. Make paper aeroplanes and see whose will fly the furthest.

64. Play balloon tennis.

65. Make rings out of paper plates. Keep the cardboard inside of kitchen towel. Now throw the rings at the cardboard and see who can get it the ring inside the cardboard inset.

66. If you have a Nerf gun set up an indoor shooting range

67. Make some Air Dry Clay and make something cool.

https://qrs.ly/19bdo5v

"4 ounces of corn starch, 4 ounces of glue, 1 tablespoons of vegetable or baby oil, 1 tablespoon of lemon juice or white vinegar... mix it all together and it is ready to go!" Source: Tutorial and video by Whatsupmoms.

68. Ball toss: Get different size buckets and put a value on each. Toss a ball into them and add up the score after 4 throws each.

69. Laser Maze. Stick tape from one door to another at angles, throughout the hallway. Get past without touching the tape.

QR video link provides you with 22 FUN activities to do

https://qrs.ly/tcbduaj

10 Science activities to do, watch the video

https://qrs.ly/bfbdugl

100 things to do when you're BORED AT HOME!

https://qrs.ly/zsbe0v4

Extracts from the book

Climate Cancer

Published in this book by permission of the publisher and author

Dave Smith

Quotes

"I've had a million dreams about the world ending...Its weird cause it feels like a movie...we are about to die if we don't change...everyone's life matters" **Billie Eilish**

Scan to see Billie and Woody's Greenpeace video on climate change, my house is on fire

https://qrs.ly/xzbdokq

Many Thanks to Greta Thunberg and all the other young activists around the world who are taking on Governments and Politician to drive forward change for a climate emergency. Now it's global, **and** she has inspired children and adults, while lobbying Politician and Governments on the need for immediate climate action.

"The eyes of all future generations are upon you. And if you choose to fail us, I say - we will never forgive you." – Greta Thunberg at the UN Climate Summit, New York, 23 September 2019

"We showed that we are united and that we, young people, are unstoppable." – Greta Thunberg at the UN Youth Climate Summit, New York City, 21 September 2019

"Future generations are growing up in a world that is being destroyed by past and current generations. No longer can Politicians be allowed to make indecisive decisions that prolong real and immediate action to avert a climate disaster. Become a climate activist today and fight for climate justice."

Children are the future and in our children we must trust. But can our children trust Governments, leaders and the adults of this world?

We all have the power to change our climate for the better, but that change needs to be started NOW. Not tomorrow or by 2050, but NOW. If it wasn't for activists like Greenpeace, Extinction Rebellion, Greta Thunberg and many more making the public aware of facts that Governments and companies have tried to hide, our earth would be in a far worse dilemma.

Every person can make a difference for our planet by:

- Only getting your energy from green providers.

- Only buy products from suppliers that are using green technology, such as delivery by electric vehicles and sustainable food sources

- Reduce huge agricultural damaging emissions (estimated between 14% to 22% of overall pollution) by changing your diet and eating less meat

- Campaign for Electric Vehicles to be available for everyone and not just the rich.

- Become a climate and environmental activist

On Friday 20th September, my youngest child joined the global school climate strike that Greta Thunberg started. That morning I walked to work so I could join my child at the strike rally. [Please note- The Department of Education did not support this, as a result my son was penalised for attending the global school strike – And this is a UK Government department – Shame on you...How can you be responsible for education when you can't even support children who are educating YOU on the danger of the climate crisis? Are you not supposed to be the Educators? Government departments do not have a clue nor are these Government departments working together to solve the climate change problem?]

My personal pledge: To use my car less and walk or cycle whenever I can. Not only is it healthier but a breath of fresh air for our planet. To become a vegetarian. [So far this is my 9th month of being a vegetarian, though occasional I succumb. My pledge to try harder and educate myself on healthy plant based eating...To encourage people to seek true scientific information and to work on stopping fossil fuel pollution.

What is your personal pledge?

Many people are now trying to do their bit, but it is difficult to change your ways. How would you get your children to school when public transport is not available, and the school is too far away to cycle to?

The dilemma that stops people from doing their bit: Sometimes you have to travel by car to your work or for business meetings. You have children to take too different clubs miles apart, you still have to go to work, and do the shopping, and make dinner for everyone returning home. Anxiety and Stress forms as you find it impossible to make the changes needed to reduce climate damage by ditching your fossil fuel car. But how can you do all of these tasks in the time allocated without a form of personal transportation? The frustration sets in, you feel overwhelmed and you sit back down and think what the fuck! What can I do? So you push climate change into the hidden part of your brain. But if you do one small thing to help your climate it's a start, right?

The Government must take the lead and make green and sustainable energy and electric transportation available for everyone and right now. People cannot be guilt-tripped into doing their bit by your current unscrupulous Government who then lack the drive and ambition to do something real other than words of, "We have declared a Climate Emergency." Governments need to be proactive and set an example.

Move to public transport and the health of people travelling on them

I read an article that the UK Government will attempt to restrict personal car journeys and increase public transportation. This was released in the midst of the coronavirus outbreak, in this instance a reliance on public transport could be flawed both on a mobility but also a health issue. Coronavirus has highlighted that close proximity of people allows the virus to spread, so it's the same for other virus like the flu. Therefore, we must maintain social distancing. Therefore, jammed packed public transport (buses, trains, underground subways etc.) can no longer be tolerated or allowed?

Who will be the ones allowed cars? The wealth or the people in power? That would be totally unacceptable by any means. What about people currently in areas where public transport is inaccessible, or they would have quite a distance to walk with their shopping? Shopping could be changed radically where people don't actual bring any shopping with them, as all shopping (food or otherwise) would be delivered by electric transportation?

Would stopping cheap flights help? In this instance I would have to agree with Michael O'Leary of Ryanair, increasing fares would only allow the rich to travel, the little people would be fucked. And that's not fair. The rich cannot have an upper-hand, we should not allow the rich to afford fossil fuel products, services or transportation when the poor cannot afford to.

What I know is that the people employ the Government. The people should have a major voice in any of these major decisions and not only at election time.

The Death of a Homeless Man

When raising money for cancer I was fortunate enough to meet Jimmy Brolly. He was a popular man that walked the streets of Derry while pushing all of his belongings in a shopping trolley. He lived on the street and sometimes in a homeless shelter. Jimmy died at 59 years of age in November 2019. He was well known around the town and many of the people in Derry raised money for his funeral.

While his death gave a stark reminder, that society needs to be doing and caring more for homeless people, it also highlighted his carbon footprint. Jimmy walked everywhere pushing his shopping trolley that contained all of his belongings. Jimmy's carbon footprint on co2 emissions was basically the air he exhaled. Yet everyone who drives a car throughout the world is polluting our atmosphere well over 4 Tonnes of co2 emissions per car per year.

The clothes and products you purchase have a co2 factor from raw source, to manufacture, to distribution, to shop, to your purchase, to your 'discarding' of that product, and finally the pollution or recycling of that product.

The above are vital points, why should the Jimmy's or the people of the world [who can't afford their own car or as many other unneeded products] have to suffer from climate change that others have caused via pollution to our planet?

Who gives others the right to pollute the planet?

Freedom does not mean that you have a right to pollute and kill others through your greedy materialistic values and ways of living.

You have no right to murder a child or an adult. So why do you think you have a right to murder your children's future on earth due to your denial or lack of action to avert a climate catastrophe of an extinction magnitude? The true polluters are those from developed countries who have taken part in our throw away culture.

How can we as Individuals make a difference to our climate?

1) Send a message to your Politician's and leaders and ask for more to be done to halt climate change.

2) DON'T vote for ANY Politician or party that does not put the CLIMATE FIRST.

3) Only purchase goods or services from shops, businesses and companies who are making a change towards a climate fix. We need change NOW not in years to come.

4) Campaign for public transport to be green. Only travel in taxis that use electric vehicles.

5) Force transport and delivery companies to use electric vehicles

6) Campaign local councils and Governments for grants to make it affordable for people to switch to fossil free vehicles.

7) Change energy providers to green sustainable energy providers. And campaign against non-sustainable energy companies.

8) Grants for households, streets, and local communities to produce their own fossil free energy. Solar, wind power etc.

9) Campaign for Businesses to ban personal fossil fuelled car travel at least once per month to start with.

10) Turn off lights and electrical appliances when not in use.

11) Take a shower instead of a bath

12) Eat less red meat and replace with a healthy plant-based diet

13) Recycle clothes and equipment

14) Recycle waste

15) Don't purchase plastic bottled water or plastic bags.

16) Do not purchase singular use plastic items. Plastic pollution is creating havoc in our environment. From manufacturing all the way to our food chain (ocean and land.) Plastic pollution is now being found in human bodies.

17) Don't purchase food items stored in unsustainable packaging.

18) Develop a shop badge of climate worthiness and only buy from shops that display their climate worthiness. (Similar to the Michelin star for food)

19) **Make a CLIMATE PLEDGE RESOLUTION – Car Free last Friday of every month within all Government, local councils and all Governmental or local authority bodies.**

20) Campaign to make your town centres vehicle free.

The world has not achieved the Paris agreement's agreed reduction in fossil fuel emissions. Global sea levels are still rising, ocean heat is still increasing, Ice sheets and glaziers are still melting. The world is experiencing droughts, fires, floods, and pollution continues to increase.

WMO (World Meteorological Organisation)

"The year 2019 concludes...is on course to be the second or third warmest year on record, according to the World Meteorological Organisation."

https://qrs.ly/cvbdocn   https://qrs.ly/qfbdokj

Other Campaigns Ideas

- Campaign local shops, businesses, taxi companies to become green.

- Campaign to stop fossil fuel car imports

- Campaign to stop production of fossil fuel vehicles IMMEDIATELY

- Campaign for more research into replacing fossil fuelled vehicles

- Campaign for sustainable foods

- Campaign for fossil free fuelled aircrafts

- Campaign for free solar panels for every household

- Campaign for your school to be more ecological friendly.

- Campaign for your school to take on board Adverse Childhood Experiences and how they can affect every child and adult in your community.

- Campaign for your local authority and Government to operate only electric vehicles

- Campaign for cheaper "to buy" Electric Vehicle.

- Campaign for environmental grants for your home in. E.g. Solar Power, Electric car purchase with major discounts.

- Brainstorm in groups or by yourself and make your own list

- Has your local council declared a climate emergency? If not campaign them to do so.

For all future school climate strikes: Everyone needs to join them.

Adults and businesses should stand by children's hard work in their attempts at saving the planet. Go on strike with the children. Now that countries are coming out of a world pandemic lock-down, you may well find that leaders will try to get you to stop such action in their quest to heal a fractured economy. However, if you listen to such requests, then you will seal the fate for your children's future. And that fate will be an extremely bleak future.

- Message to the parent and child, do not allow any school to force you to stay at school when on climate strike.
- Message to the parent, make sure your child is not penalised by attending climate strikes. Support your child's strike and attend yourself whenever possible.
- Message to the Education board and school, do the right thing and support the school children's climate strike action. After all you expect parents and children to support you when on strike.

Fighting Cancer, Human and Climate

I like many others have had friends and family members suffer and die through distinct types of cancer. [I have used the term climate cancer because, a) we all loathe this curse of a disease and b) by referring to climate as cancer, perhaps we will all realise how dangerous climate change is and do something personal about it now and c) Climate change is really a cancerous growth caused by humans to infect our atmosphere, our planet, ourselves and other life forms.] And they saved as previously outlined 77 thousand lives because of pollution reductions in China.

As we are all united to fight cancer, we must all be unified to fight for climate justice for the future of your children's existence. You can no longer accept what your generation has done to the world's climate. As is in a court of law you can no longer claim ignorance as a means of defence.

Climate change is really "Climate Cancer," it is destroying the lungs of our planet (the trees and the air we breathe), melting ice caps and glaciers affecting our sea levels and ocean currents (our arteries), earth is slowing dying reducing human sustainability (our heart.)

Even our food chain is becoming polluted, they have found micro plastics in the building block of life (Plankton), in the intestines of fish, and within birds and other animals that feed on fish products. Did you know that cows, sheep and chickens are eating particles of plastic items discarded from our throw away culture and their feed and feed bags? This now affects every person in society and throughout the world in some form or another.

Likewise, climate cancer is human created, and every one of us has the power to change this perilous pathway that we are on. We all have an opportunity to play a personal role in slowing down the damage and easing human suffering while providing earth with a chance to heal itself. Climate cancer will continue to grow and spread, it will keep doing this, unless we radically change our PERSONAL way of life.

Human Heath before Human wealth

Trump and many other world leaders are ignoring scientists and proven statistics towards the consequences of climate damage. Are they that naïve or just masquerading as Hitler's?

Trump has obscene wealth, his wealth will secure his family a place in a world that runs on a financial system, assuming that wealth will still count in fifty years' time? The poor as usual will pay the price for the damage that greedy corporations, individuals and denying Governments have done to our planet. Done via greed and a clamber to be the richest and most powerful in the world.

The definition of a scumbag: A person who is dishonest, contemptible, undesirable or sleazy. Politician and Governments who put the overall welfare of our planet as second to greed and financial wealth fit this description to a tee.

I have never believed in name calling or labelling. However, we really need to call it by what it is. As such I have broken my naming calling belief. We need to portray such Governments and Politician for what they really have portrayed themselves as, and that's 'SCUMBAGS'

- Was Hitler a scumbag?

- Was Hitler mad?

- Was Hitler a monster?

Hitler was responsible for the murder, genocide and culling of tens of millions of people around the globe. If he hadn't been stopped, then our world today would be a worse place to live.

We cannot allow Politician and Governments to commit 'climate genocide' when they already knew about climate change and subsequent climate damage for over one hundred years.

While the atrocities of what Hitler did during WW1 and WW2 is utterly disgraceful, inhumane and cowardly, the lack of what our Governments and officials are doing towards halting climate damage will be far worse. The result of this ignorance is not acceptable and ultimately such officials should be held responsible for the cull of tens of millions of people and billions of other earth's species.

It was reported in January 2020 that the UK Government will be sued because of its stupidity in approving the biggest gas power station in Europe. The UK Government overruled climate objections and spearheaded this planned production facility past normal channels of planning. The UK Government ignored its own countries agreed reduction in co2 production and emissions to build this factory of destruction. This results from scumbag Politician and a Government with a two faced climate agenda.

In an interview with Claire Perry regarding Prime Minister Johnson and climate change, *'Johnson has also admitted to me that he doesn't really understand it. He doesn't really get it.'* Prime Minister Johnson contracted COVID-19 and is now out of intensive care, many people rallied around and said that they would pray for his recovery. Regardless of any feeling that people have towards his handling of the UK Government, no one wants any person throughout the world to die from this virus. History will surly dictate who did what and was it soon enough or could there have been more done? What we don't want is history telling your grandchildren that not enough was done soon enough to stop climate cancer from killing billions of people.

Human Health should always come before human wealth.

False and Hidden statistics: they blame Developing countries for producing vast co2 emissions and pollutions, this is done not by that countries inhabitants. It's done by the developed countries need for cheap labour for the production of goods coming back into these developed countries. Thereby maximising the sales and profits of those corporations.

This is what I call the 'false and hidden statistics' of the USA, UK, Europe and other developed countries. They get other countries to mass produce their goods utilising child & cheap labour while increasing that countries co2 emissions and other pollutions. In reality if the 'goods' were all produced in the developed countries then their co2 emissions would be obscenely high.

Leaders around the world are quick on the band wagon at posting blame towards China for the damage that they are doing to the world's climate. Now China has come under threat by the USA president Trump and some other countries for the blame for the Coronavirus.

First, China's vast amounts of pollution is a direct result of developed countries demand for products to be exported from china to other countries. In fact if the countries ordering products from China were to manufacture these products in their own country then their co2 and pollution figures would explode while Chinas would fall drastically.

The USA's emissions per person drastically exceeds those of china's emissions per person. Don't let Governments provide you with misleading statistics. China has a far higher population therefore their total country emissions should naturally be higher.

Therefore, if China was on the same level playing field as other developed countries then it would be safe to assume that their populations should have gas guzzling vehicles, enormous homes, and all the other fancy gadgets that Americans and others in developed countries have. Right?

I want to apologise, as there may be some repetition of facts and statements throughout this book, but I believe that they are necessary to plant a seed in your brain. That seed hopefully will germinate and grow into a motivational journey that will spearhead you to do some of your own research and become a person with an addiction for knowledge and action to halt climate change. Please join other activist's on a common pathway towards halting climate change, for climate justice needs you, and so does your children's future.

Below are extracts from newspapers **along with**

The author's sometimes sarcastic but sadly true comments

The Independent quoted Trump as:

"Speaking at a press conference before departing the World Economic Forum, the American president suggested the 17-year-old Swede "ought to focus on" other countries than the US, which he insisted was "clean and beautiful" and where "everything is good...Our numbers are very good, our environmental numbers..."

Source: https://www.independent.co.uk/news/world/europe/trump-greta-thunberg-davos-speech-climate-change-time-magazine-world-economic-forum-a9296481.html

Actual fact: The USA beats China and India on co2 emissions if compared against "per capita" or is it the fact that Greta is a girl and teenager that upsets Trump? How dare anyone tell the president of the United States of America that he is wrong?

Moreover, the USA and their corporations build factories in China and India to produce goods for the USA. So the pollution and co2 emissions from such industries in China and India really belong to the USA. Get your facts right Mr President.

BT.COM quoted:

US Treasury Secretary Steven Mnuchin has said Swedish climate activist Greta Thunberg is in no position to give economic advice until she goes to college and comes out with an economics degree.

https://home.bt.com/news/world-news/us-treasury-secretary-tells-greta-thunberg-to-go-to-college-and-get-a-degree-11364427168720

What an idiot Steven Mnuchin is, does he really believe that no one has any right to point out undeniable facts backed up by science, statistics and what can be seen happening to our Earth today, unless they have a college degree? Is he saying that everyone on earth who does not have a college degree is worthless?

Russia

Sad but true: According to the Kremlin website it has recognised that global heating is a problem. However they deny that climate damage is caused by humans and they have stated that it has economic benefits for their nation.

Here we can see that some countries who could be better off are planning to use climate damage for their own benefit and fuck everyone else.

Research: I researched the above from Kremlin website and The Guardian newspaper "Russia announces plan to use the advantages of climate change.

Oxfam project:

"Britons reach Africans annual carbon emissions in just two weeks." This was a report from an Oxfam project as reported in the guardian newspaper.

Britons and other developed countries and their populations are destroying our planet at the expense of countries less advanced.

When will people wake up and realise that they cannot keep spending money on crap products that they really don't need? When will people realise that we cannot pollute our atmosphere with co2 and other contaminants?

Become Responsible:

You cannot sit back and allow the Government to take all the flack.

- Each person needs to **become an activist**.

- Each person needs to accept their own responsibility for polluting the planet and make amends and change.

- Each person has the power to reduce their own co2 emissions, pollution and product wastefulness.

If you want to keep a similar lifestyle, then these four problems must be resolved first and with a matter of immediate urgency.

1. Sustainable and renewable energy production.

2. Fossil fuel free vehicles and aircraft, operating on sustainable energy.

3. A reduction in waste and product manufacturing and recycle more.

4. Reduction in commercial farming with a move towards plant based food production.

Without Activist's
Our world today would be a worse place!

- Human rights activists have changed the world for the better

- Environmental activists have change the world for the better

- Woman's rights activist have changed the world for the better

- Activists fighting poverty have changed the world for the better

- Activists fighting child abuse have changed the world for the better

- Activists fighting domestic violence laws have changed the world for the better

- Activists fighting for bio-diversity rights of other species are changing the world for the better

- Activists fighting for charities (charities are needed because our Politician's and Governments have let the people down...a financial system and the Government's relationship with corporations are more important than everything else. We need a radical change, and we need it NOW)

- Activists fighting for a destruction to the trafficking and paedophile networks are changing the world for the better

Do you therefore think we can allow Politician's and Governments away with creating climate genocide on a massive scale that will affect earth and every species on it?

I think not! Become a Climate Activist today.

Words of doom and gloom are all around us, how can we be resilient?

Every day we are bombarded by climate damage, climate disasters, famine, poverty and abuse and so forth. It can become overwhelming. So much so that fear, depression and a lack of not knowing what one can do to avert these impending disasters overcomes us.

To become resilient, you cannot let yourself become overwhelmed.

Therefore, resilience is the power within you to make a change for the better. You can multitask... you can fight personal trauma and grief...you can fight for your children's future. **Resilience is within you, it only needs awakened.**

Don't let the doom and gloom get you down, pick one area of climate damage and make a change for the better. At least you are trying. And trying is resilience.

Extract from the DeadS Bible *"You will not be judged on your death bed by the wealth, fame or power that you have amassed, you cannot take these with you when you die. You will be judged purely on the kindness and goodness that your life has marked on earth. All species are equal, your job is to create a world where peace, harmony, equality among all exists. You are all brother, sisters and children of the infinite universe, you all bleed the same blood, your planet is sacred to you and too many other species look after it wisely."*

When you die, you will leave an impending disaster for future generations. Now is your time to make a stand and fight for climate justice before it really is too late for the children of the future.

A Climate Emergency means just that! It's an EMERGENCY! It's not a rhetoric talk without emergency action.

I read an article in the Guardian Newspaper by Bill McKibben. He demonstrated that while Trump was a climate denier the American people elected him. While Canada was all for helping the climate heal and they believed that the climate crisis is real. But still the Canadian Government is set to approve a huge new tar sands mine, this will pour carbon into the atmosphere all the way past the 2060s.

Who are the biggest Idiots Trump or the Canadian Government? However it also makes you wonder how Trump can get elected by the American people when he thinks climate change is a hoax, surely the American people are not that stupid?

The above story is both despair and hypocrisy at its highest level within countries.

Extract from the Extinction Rebellion Video: *"We are facing an unprecedented global emergency. Life on Earth is in crisis: scientists agree we have entered a period of abrupt climate breakdown, and we are in the midst of a mass extinction of our own making. ,"*

https://qrs.ly/xabbp2t

Kids Climate Videos, great for Adults too

Below is a QR link to a **NASA kid's video explaining what the difference between Climate and Weather**? Explained in a child's way. But suitable for adults and children.

https://qrs.ly/3ebbog6

The debate and denial about climate change needs to end NOW. We need Solutions, and most solutions currently exist and are available to roll out and implement.

Bill Nye narrates this short film on the basics of climate change.

https://qrs.ly/4pbbxpg

The Shit affect

Trump and his administration have received immense amounts of funding from these industries. Why do you think Trump is playing the idiot and denial cap? His statement at a rally makes it crystal clear what kind of leader he is. **"It's freezing... where is global warming...its freezing here"**

https://qrs.ly/8lbbog2

Scan above QR code to listen to Trump saying the above words of stupidity. Trump is an exceptional businessman, and he has made billions of dollars of the back of the little people. But when it comes to being a world leader he is nothing but an IDIOT-1 whose party is being funded by the coal and oil companies.

On the 4th March they announced that a prominent scientific paper has retracted its original study, the USA administration previously cited this in its denial of climate change. The study previously claimed that climate change was because of solar cycles rather than human activity. In a statement today scientific reports said that this was inaccurate. This is another nail in the coffin for deniers who misused this information, ask yourself for what gain?

Humans have achieved fantastic innovations and have come a long way since the Stone Age. However this has come at a grave cost to humans and our planet.

"Never before has man had such a great capacity to control his own environment, to end hunger, poverty and disease, to banish illiteracy and human misery. We have the power to make the best

generation of mankind in the history of the world." **John F. Kennedy**

"The warnings about global warming have been extremely clear for a long time. We are facing a global climate crisis. It is deepening. We are entering a period of consequences." **Al Gore**

"...Its freezing...We want more global warming...Its freezing..." **Donald Trump**

The Lancet Commission report on Health and Climate Change says that *"the threat to human health from climate change is so great that it could undermine the last fifty years of gains in development and global health... Measures to combat climate change could bring health benefits by reducing pollution. Air pollution is responsible for 30,000 excess deaths each year in the UK and seven million worldwide."* Is this the hidden agenda for Governments around the world, to curb the increasing world's population by denial? When I was born the world population was 2.8 billion. In February 2020 the world's population is 7.8 billion. An increase of more than 3 times in the space of sixty years.

It has been reported that a Government USA official has been inserting misleading language about climate change into the agencies reports. Mr. Goklany is accused of inserting misleading interpretations of climate science. With Government officials lying through their teeth. Trump and his administration are destroying our planet.

I want to introduce you to the "Shit effect". The "Shit effect" is for all the deniers of Climate pollution.

To the deniers, visualise that you are laying in a hot bath and gently washing your body. I come along with excrement in tow, how much animal and human shit do I have to drop into your hot relaxing bath before you leap out shouting and screaming in disgust and fear for your health? One minuscule bit of polluting poo? A spoonful of polluting poo? What would it take to get you to jump out of that bath?

That's exactly what you are doing to our atmosphere. CO_2 and all the other pollutants are invading our atmosphere, mother earth and the greenhouse effect cannot heal from that massive additional pollution that humans are discarding into the atmosphere. In return mother earth cannot save us from this human made climate cancer. Your God is not coming to save you either. But humans can save mother earth and humans can save humans. The ball is in our court, is it Health before wealth or is it business as normal after COVID-19. This pandemic is a warning sign, so Governments of the world do the right thing and change how we life, before it's too late.

"Exposure to nitrogen dioxide, nitrogen oxide, sulphur dioxide, and fine particulate matter were positively associated with a risk of lung cancer. Occupational exposure to air pollution among professional drivers significantly increased the incidence and mortality of lung cancer." The Authors. Thoracic Cancer published by Tianjin Lung Cancer Institute and Wiley Publishing Asia Pty Ltd.

Smoking - Trump - Cows and lots more

Tobacco smoking is "slow and assisted suicide." In the UK the Suicide act clarifies that "assisted suicide" is illegal. So ask yourself one question, why do the UK Government still allow tobacco companies to assist in the murder of innocent people? This assisted suicide by tobacco companies should see every director of these companies in jail.

Report by WHO, *"About 7 million people per year die from air pollution-related diseases. These include stroke and heart disease, respiratory illness and cancers. Many other harmful air pollutants also damage the climate. Fine particles of black carbon (soot) from diesel and biomass combustion and ground level ozone are leading examples. Reducing air pollution would save lives and help slow the pace of near-term climate change."*

"Saving our planet, lifting people out of poverty, advancing economic growth... these are one and the same fight. We must connect the dots between climate change, water scarcity, energy shortages, global health, food security, and women's empowerment. Solutions to one problem must be solutions for all."
– Ban Ki-moon

In a science report issued in 1912 *[Science Notes and News" section of The Rodney and Otamatea Times, published Wednesday, Aug. 14, 1912.New Zealand. Scientists reported these facts]* it outlined that fossil fuel use will create a catastrophic greenhouse effect with the temperatures of earth rising to unacceptable levels within the next 100 years [and that report has now come true]. Yet despite this warning and thousands of other warnings since then, Governments and Politicians have increased co2 and other greenhouse gases production and emissions at a rate unjustifiable to that what was stated and outlined in the 1912 report. Moreover, countries have miserably failed to meet emission deadlines as set by the Paris agreement (Signed in 2016, USA withdrew from this agreement in 2019 because Trump stated it will affect the financial viability of businesses in the USA).

On the 19th February 2020 the USA Republican Party and President Trump have mandated the continued use of fossil fuels... further fuelling earth's extinction. Under their mandate your children and their children will not have a future.

Scan the QR image below to listen to a national geographic video based In Appalachia, coal companies blow the tops off of mountains to get at the coal. The damage this does to the surrounding environment and water supply is devastating.

https://qrs.ly/ypbboo5

People laugh when they hear how cows are damaging our climate with their farts. Scan the QR image below to see a video that shows you in actual terms how cows are contributing to global warming. At first when I saw this video I thought it was unethical of what was happening to these cows, but then I thought well it's better than ending up as steaks on a table. Or for testing on makeup, right? I'm still not sure.

https://qrs.ly/yibbosn

Simple math's: 1.5 billion cows x 50 gallon bags of methane produced per day = 75 billion gallons of methane per day x 20 (20 times more potent than co2) = 1,500 billion gallon bags. Homework: Now do your own research and see what those gallon bags equate to in methane emissions. Staggering is it not?

One reason Trump has earned his IDIOT-1 title is because of his statement below. How can a president be so stupid?

Trump in front of a rally: *"It is supposed to be 70 degrees here today, it's freezing. Speaking of global warming, where is global warming? We need some global warming. It's freezing... It's time to put America first, and that includes a promise to cancel billions in climate change spending. Our plan will end the EPA."*

Al Gore, *"The next generation, will be justified at looking back at us and asking, WHAT WERE YOU THINKING? COULD YOU NOT HEAR WHAT THE SCIENTISTS WHERE SAYING? COULD YOU NOT HEAR AND SEE WHAT MOTHER NATURE WAS SCREAMING AT YOU?*

Scan QR Code below to see Trump and Al Gore say the above words:

https://qrs.ly/8lbbog2

Donald Trump will be 74 years of age on 14th June 2020. The life expectancy for a male born in 1946 in the USA is 78 years of age. In theory he has 4 years remaining on earth. He does not care about your children's future. His children and family have billions of dollars that will secure them a place in a world that is being destroyed at the hands of his greed. His wealth was made from the backs of the little people. He also stated that he would use some of his wealth to build a wall between the USA and Mexico. Trump is for destruction at all levels. He is selfish and uncaring person. Why could he not use all of his wealth to help end poverty or homelessness?

"Nobody on this planet is going to be untouched by the impacts of climate change." **Rajendra K. Pachauri**

"We cannot solve our problems with the same thinking we used when we created them." **Albert Einstein**

"How could I look my grandchildren in the eye and say I knew what was happening to the world and did nothing." **David Attenborough.**

It is one small step to declare a 'Climate Emergency' but the monumental step is treating it as an emergency. An emergency requires immediate action. Can you imagine being taken to hospital with a life-threatening emergency and the doctors and nurses stand over you looking, planning, going for a cup of coffee, coming back again and discussing what they should do next? If they did, you would be dead. Likewise, the climate emergency needs immediate action and a drastic change, otherwise your planet will be dead.

"There are risks and costs to action. But they are far less than the long-range risks of comfortable inaction.

One person can make a difference, and everyone should try.

The world is very different now. For man holds in his mortal hands the power to abolish all forms of human poverty, and all forms of human life." **John F. Kennedy.**

"The Earth is not dying-it is being killed. And the people who are killing it have names and addresses." **Utah Phillips.**

If you do nothing now, then 2050 will face the biggest clamber for survival and civil war's involving all of humankind. It's a hopeless horizon that will witness the destruction of all living things on earth. That's your children's future.

HOPE exists, but it requires now action to facilitate a Hope towards a Future for your children. **Become a climate activist, your children and planet NEEDS YOU.**

There is a lot of talk about **Net Zero**, but Net Zero is not the ultimate solution. Zero emissions is the correct and best solution for our future. Net Zero, is like allowing smokers in a room filled with trees. However, the smoke will still kill you. Net Zero is the cop out version of Governments who lack any resourcefulness or 'balls' to do the right thing and that's to stop pollution and fossil fuel burning at any cost.

Scan the QR below to see an explanation of net zero.

https://qrs.ly/c2bbp11

There is no doubt that the climate emergency will devour lives. Climate deniers will make sure of that. The battle to save humanity and earth will without a certain of doubt begin sooner than what we think. In the light of human displacement already occurring around the world today as a result of poverty, malnutrition, droughts, famines and land loss the fight to stay alive will become a humanitarian's nightmare.

We need to convince people of the emergency not only by words but with emergency tactics of action. On the 2nd of March 2020, ninety seven Barclay's Bank Branches throughout the UK were kept closed by Greenpeace activist. Greenpeace claims that Barclay's is one of the largest funders of fossil fuels in Europe.

Sustainable development goals

https://qrs.ly/jrbdo0d

The facts you need to know about the Climate Emergency:

https://qrs.ly/zcbdo0g

Climate Cancer 2020
Together we can make a stand and fight for climate justice.
Or
We can watch it disintegrate in front of us.

Doctors or Surgeons will not do the first response to resolving climate cancer, but rather by a cooperation involving billions of innocent people. All standing together in civil disobedience and solidarity to fight Politician's, leaders and Governments who fail to act as if it's not an emergency. Listen to Great Thunberg in the video below.

https://qrs.ly/t4bdoap

"At first when I heard about climate change, I was a climate denier. I didn't think it was happening. Because if there really was an existential crisis like that, that would threaten our civilisation, we wouldn't be focusing on anything else." **Greta Thunberg.**

Support the school strikes. Create a climate workers strike. DO SOMETHING! We cannot leave it to our children to fix the mess that ours and past generations have created. Stand by, and be with the children, make your family voice heard.

School Children go on strike

https://qrs.ly/1hbdo5z

School Strikes

https://qrs.ly/xnbdo9d

Climate Cancer

- The human body is a complex system made from millions of cells.

- Earth is a complex home created for the survival of all living things.

The greenhouse effect sustains life on earth and when it is effected by excess human harmful co2 emissions, then this orderly process breaks down and Climate Cancer begins.

Our atmosphere is becoming polluted with co2 emissions, this is a cancerous growth as it has major affects for human health, and earth's ability to sustain life. This unnatural greenhouse growth affects earth, temperature rises which causes ice caps and glaciers to melt which raises sea water levels, which claims land masses, which in turns dissipates people and destroys vast land areas making them inhabitable. Furthermore, unnatural change affects weather and creates droughts, heatwaves, floods, and extreme weather storms.

The major question is, "are humans responsible for earth's cancerous growth?" The answer is without a doubt and sadly "yes" humans are fully responsible for what they have done to your planet. But humans have the power to change and amend their ways before our climate changes irreversibly and life on earth becomes uncertain.

Climate Cancer, can be cured, but it will take a drastic change to the way we life today. Governments around the world are making some effort towards change, but not adequate or quick enough. Governments are way behind the agreement to reduce co2 emissions as per the Paris Agreement. So much so that our climate damage is speeding up and will surpass the predicted damage.

Climate Cancer can be stopped, but first you need to make some drastic life changing choices. If you don't then it's your children that will suffer. Will you be selfish? Or will you help save your children?

Now Is the Time for action. If the word "Cancer with Climate" does not make you stop, think and realise how you have been conditioned and brainwashed by money-oriented goals, then there is no hope for the current pathway of humanity. As such you shall have inescapably sealed the fate for your children and their generation's future.

The president of the USA Donald Trump in a speech belittled every scientist in the world that has provided evidence about the climate emergency when he stated, "It's Freezing here, where is the global warming...its freezing here...we want some global warming...its freezing." But seriously what a "beep...beep" IDIOT-1 he is.

"For way too long, the politicians and the people in power have gotten away with not doing anything to fight the climate crisis, but we will make sure that they will not get away with it any longer. We are striking because we have done our homework and they have not." **Greta Thunberg.**

Research and Climate Videos

17 Goals to Transform Our World

The Sustainable Development Goals are a call for action by all countries – poor, rich and middle-income – to promote prosperity while protecting the planet. They recognise that ending poverty must go hand-in-hand with strategies that build economic growth and address a range of social needs including education, health, social protection, and job opportunities, while tackling climate change and environmental protection.

https://qrs.ly/xgbd4dd

What's the difference between weather and climate?

NASA Kids

https://qrs.ly/1vbd4e2

Climate Change is a real and serious issue. In this video Bill Nye, the Science Guy, explains what causes climate change, how it affects our planet, why we need to act promptly to mitigate its effects, and how each of us can contribute to a solution.

https://qrs.ly/obbd4e8

Informed debate on energy and climate change - Information

https://qrs.ly/41bd4ee

Famed scientist and educator Bill Nye is an outspoken advocate for climate change action. Through elections and scientific innovation, The Science Guy sees a world where climate denialism dies out.

https://qrs.ly/zebd4en

CLIMATE 101 with BILL NYE as he shows the greenhouse effect in 2 glass jars

https://qrs.ly/4pbbxpg

RACING EXTINCTION https://qrs.ly/bkbd4es

Displacement: Fleeing climate change -- the real environmental disaster | DW Documentary

https://qrs.ly/cibd4gv

The number of people fleeing war, persecution and conflict exceeded 70 million in 2018 - the highest level that UNHCR has seen in its almost 70 years. UNHCR reports on the state of force displacement. Scan the QR image below to view.

https://qrs.ly/5tbd4h2

Dr David Cantor, Director of the University of London's Refugee Law Initiative, gives a brief introduction to the issues surrounding refugees who have been displaced from their homes because of global warming or natural disasters.

https://qrs.ly/15bd4h9

National Geographic, What causes climate change (also known as global warming)? And what are the effects of climate change? Learn the human impact and consequences of climate change for the environment, and our lives.

It Causes, Asthma, Lung cancer and heart disease

https://qrs.ly/a1bd4hn

After over three decades, the public is finally beginning to grasp what a serious threat global warming poses. What's missing from the climate conversation now is a plausible narrative about how we might parry this threat. Drawing on ideas from his recently published book, Under the Influence: Putting Peer Pressure to Work, Robert Frank explains why our ability to tap the prodigious power of behavioural contagion may make the path forward less daunting than many think. Recorded on 1/27/2020. (One hour 21 mins long)

https://qrs.ly/yubd4hw

Matt Miltonberger, Matt's first full animated info-graphic, 4 months of researching, calculating, writing, illustrating, animating, and editing.
Climate change is a real and serious issue. **Brilliant & creative work.**

https://qrs.ly/sgbd4i4

We could get a third of the way to our climate change goals with no technology at all. All we need is to turn to the power of nature. Here are three natural strategies that could help us solve the climate crisis.

https://qrs.ly/m4bd4id

Reducing your carbon footprint just got easier. This video uses animations and humour to teach people how they can help prevent global warming. This is just one of the free educational products available in the "Climate Insights 101" series. Created by the Pacific Institute for Climate Solutions (PICS) -- a collaboration of British Columbia's four research intensive universities.

https://qrs.ly/8ibd4is

Cambridge University, Forests burn, glaciers melt and one million species face extinction. Can we humans save the planet from ourselves? In a recent film, alumni **Sir David Attenborough and Dr Jane Goodall DBE**, and leading Cambridge University researchers, talk about the urgency of the climate crisis – and some solutions that will take us towards zero carbon.

If we are to avoid climate disaster we must sharply reduce our carbon dioxide emissions starting today – but how? Cambridge researchers describe their work on generating and storing renewable energy, reducing energy consumption, understanding the impact of climate policies, and probing how we can each reduce our environmental impact.

https://qrs.ly/8gbd4iz

Duncan Stewart: "Climate Change - Causes, Consequences and Mitigation Solutions" | Talks at Google

Tune in to hear from award-winning architect and environmentalist Duncan Stewart in this talk on the challenges posed by greenhouse gas emissions to Earth's climate system, its affects to our young generation's future, along with affects to biodiversity, and what we can do about it.

https://qrs.ly/4vbd4j3

Electric aeroplanes

ALICE, All Electric – All Ready
Meet Alice, the world's first all-electric commuter aircraft, built to make air travel affordable and sustainable.

https://qrs.ly/iqbd4j6

Another Commercial Air company (Harbour Air Seaplanes) proposes to retrofit all of their commercial island hopper planes.

Harbour Air Seaplanes
@HarbourAirLtd

"The day the electric aviation age started..."

Thank you to our amazing maintenance team and our partners at @Magnix for bringing this project to life

We're still buzzing with excitement and this is just the beginning - it's only going to go up from here #ePlane

161   8:08 PM - Dec 11, 2019 · Harbour Air Seaplanes / Westcoast Air

As you can see from the above two stories electric commercial flights are possible and doable now. What we want is major investment and innovation to make this a reality for all aircraft manufacturing.

Extract from the MET office the Science behind Climate Change

https://qrs.ly/svbd4nt

https://qrs.ly/oobd4pv

Climate Science

The science is clear: climate change is happening. We are the cause. We need to act now.

https://qrs.ly/71bd4q5

Zero Waste

Try to become a Zero Waste family or as near as is possible. Especially under the COVID-19 circumstances. You should stay safe at all times even if it means compromising your Zero waste goals.

Lauren Singer is an Environmental Studies graduate from NYU and former Sustainability Manager watch her inspiring TED talk below.

https://qrs.ly/rubbobm

Extracts from the book

Missing in Paris

Published in this book by permission of the publisher and author

True Story, Missing People, & Mental Health

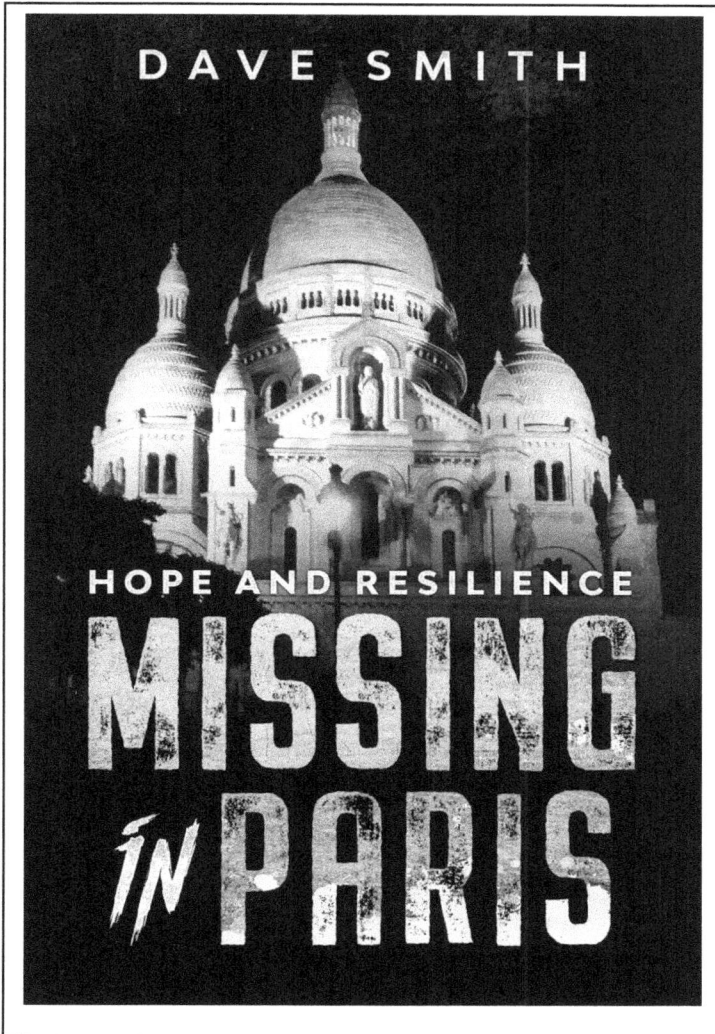

DAVE SMITH

HOPE AND RESILIENCE

MISSING IN PARIS

Extracts from the story:

...The past cannot be changed, but your future mental health can learn and heal from events in the past. Each person has the ability to reshape what has happened to them and to forge a brighter future.

...This book only touches on the trauma that Sorcha and her family faced and endured on her disappearance. A family traumatised want only one thing, they want their child (regardless of age) back home safe and sound.

...The story follows the path of Mario the "Searcher" and the search for the missing teenager. While it was like searching for 'a needle in a haystack', it was engulfed in many facets of understanding oneself, and embracing the journeys trials and tribulations while attempting to care for one's own mental health...

... Christina's phone rang, she answered it and continued to walk around the room, nodding her head in acknowledgement of what was being said. I could see the blood drain from her face. Soon a sense of loss became the birth of her crumbling body towards the slouch of despair as she sat down on the sofa.

...With tears in her eyes she put her hands to the side of her face. Christina then said, "Sorcha has gone missing."

...You hear about missing children and teenagers regularly but you never think it will be one from your family, do you?

...At this stage they did not understand what had happened to Sorcha, and what was the reasoning behind her disappearance?

... Each night before Mario went to bed, he revised his map and planned next day's tasks. What areas he was going to cover, what churches and hostels he would visit. ..

...Each morning began with Hope and each night ended with despair.

Mental Health Wellbeing

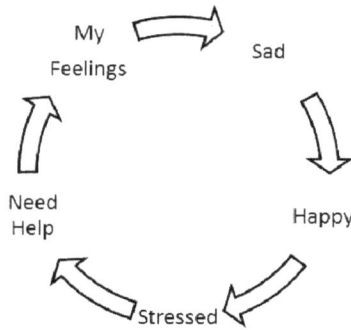

Billie Eilish's words on mental health

*"It doesn't make you weak to ask for help...
It doesn't make you weak to ask for a friend to go see a therapist."*

The other extracts below from the book 'Missing in Paris' focus on mental health and missing children and adults throughout the world.

Celebrities are now coming forward and making their mental health issues known. This in its own right is assisting in breaking the stigma and the old tradition of not talking about such things outside of the home or family. Now it's bang right out there in the open, where it should be. Workplaces are becoming more aware and by law businesses are becoming more of an informed and concerned workplace towards employees with mental health issues.

It's fantastic to see programmes of wellbeing being introduced into many workplaces, like mindfulness, meditation, healthy eating and exercise. All are proven to help reduce stress and depression.

Ruby Wax is a loud, funny woman -- who spent much of her comedy career battling depression in silence. Now her work blends mental health advocacy and laughs. [Extract from Ruby's Ted Talks]

We all sure need more humour in our lives. In this short video Ruby touches the subject head on, but in a funny and informative way. It reclassifies the stigma in people who suffer from depression and mental health issues. Today, more and more people are coming on board with the realisation that the brain is another organ that can suffer from health issues. There is nothing to be ashamed about. Mental health is like any other illness, if it needs treated then let's get on board and arrange the infrastructure to get people well again.

After all, if someone has a heart condition or cancer we look for cures. Mental health issues are present in almost every person. What separates one person displaying a mental health issue and another not, can be due to trauma, adversity, stress and toxic stress in their lives. However, some children are more adaptable and form resilience from their childhood trauma. It is further noted that a traumatised child who has one significant other that they can turn to for advice and to be there for them will act as a major form of resilience to that child

Furthermore, Ruby mentions in her video about how her mother would act in certain circumstances and this would inevitably pass mental health issues onto Ruby. The positive point of knowing that childhood experiences can shape you for better or worse is that they can also make you aware of why you are acting the way you are. And with this knowledge comes the ability to free yourself from the negative aspects of your upbringing and understand your mental health and how you can adapt from adversity or trauma to lead a fulfilling life.

Scan the QR code below to be enlightened and to have a laugh at a sad situation that can be turned around for the better.

https://qrs.ly/4qa1z0k

The voices in my head, Eleanor Longden

To all appearances, Eleanor Longden was just like every other student, heading to college full of promise and without a care in the world. That was until the voices in her head started talking... these internal narrators became increasingly antagonistic and dictatorial, turning her life into a living nightmare. Diagnosed with schizophrenia, hospitalised, drugged, Longden was discarded by a system that didn't know how to help her. Longden tells the moving tale of her years-long journey back to mental health, and makes the case that it was through learning to listen to her voices that she was able to survive.

https://qrs.ly/pua1yyc

Teen Brain Development

NIDA explores in this video the intriguing similarities between the processes of brain development and computer programming. The analogy helps us understand why toxic environmental factors like drugs, bullying, or lack of sleep can have such a long-lasting impact on a teenager's life and can be used to empower your children or students with information they need make better decisions. Extract from NDA]

https://qrs.ly/c7a1xf1

A Teenager's Brain is still developing, something that most adults forget. Our institutions (schools, police, and courts) sometimes take a dogmatic view of a teenager, when in fact studies have proven that a teenager's brain is still developing right up to mid or late twenties. This can have severe consequences on how the teenager will deal with problems that can occur in their life such as, relationships, peer, school, religious pressures and risk taking.

Teenagers break the rules because their immature brains aren't wired to properly respond to reward or punishment.

Researchers have discovered that the Adolescent brain is less likely to respond to punishments and incentives because their brains are still configuring themselves and are not yet fully developed.

Most parents and teachers can easily see that? It's almost impossible to get teenagers to focus on what you want them to do regardless of how you try to make them do what they ask.

Therefore, you need to change your methods of getting a child to respond, make it fun and interesting and mitigate a level of risk taking in the approach to the teenagers learning (such as public speaking in the class etc.)

Scan the QR code below to watch Dr Siegel's hand model describing the brain.

https://qrs.ly/ypa3pzm

Adverse Childhood Experiences (ACE's)

The Northern Ireland ACE Animation forms the basis of raising awareness of adverse childhood experiences in Northern Ireland and how you can be the change to support children, their families or adults impacted by childhood adversity.

https://qrs.ly/hw9ztik

Go to missinginparis.com and you can complete an online ACE survey.

Samaritans

If you need to talk with someone to help with your thoughts, issues or concerns. Call the Samaritans now, don't wait.

It's late, but we're waiting for your call. Whatever you're going through, a Samaritan will face it with you. We're here 24 hours a day, 365 days a year.

Call 116 123 for free

https://www.childline.org.uk/

Call Free from the UK

0800 1111

https://www.barnardos.ie

Barnardo's mission is to help transform children's lives through our services; support parents; and challenge society where it fails our children.

Missing People

HAVE YOU SEEN LEAH?

https://qrs.ly/3na3pxe

Leah disappeared on February 15th 2109 at age 19, in Milton Keynes, on her walk to work. She was last seen on Buzzacott Lane, Furzton, at about 8.15am wearing a black coat, skinny black jeans and Converse.

Leah's mum Claire made an emotional appeal and further said on the 22nd of February, 'Whatever it is that has caused you to run away, please let us help or fix it.' Claire also told everyone that

On the 25th May 2019, Chief Inspector Neil Kentish. Made the following statement, "I would like to take this opportunity to remind people of Leah's appearance; she is white, slim, with below shoulder length brown hair and sometimes wears glasses...I still believe that someone, somewhere, has a vital piece of information which will help us find Leah. If you have, and for whatever reason you haven't already come forward, I would urge you to think of Leah's family and contact the police."

The teenager's parents Claire and John Croucher said "each day getting up is the hardest thing they do... every day Leah is gone is heart-breaking she is our beautiful, wonderful daughter...but HOPE keeps them going."

Anyone with any information on Leah should contact police on 101 quoting Thames Valley Police reference 4319 004 9929

Alternatively, contact Crime stoppers anonymously on 0800 555 111 or through their online anonymous form at www.crimestoppers-uk.org. No personal details are taken, calls cannot be traced or recorded and you will not go to court.

MissingPeople.org.uk

Scan the QR code to be taken to the Missing People website.

https://qrs.ly/4ka28yb

If we all take a few moments to view photos of the missing, then perhaps you could find a missing person on your travels. The missing need all the help they can get.

MissingInParis.com

Scan the QR code below, this will take you to the Missing in Paris website. It hosts web-pages from missing people from around the world. So if you are in holiday in USA, Spain, France, Holland, etc., check the website out, look at some of the missing people's photographs. And you might just help find someone and save a life. All it takes is two minutes of your time. Please do your bit. **Please Help Find Me.**

https://qrs.ly/7da2bhh

Extracts from the Story Lyrics range of books

...Story Lyrics was born from an idea to empower young people and adults... to free you from your everyday rituals, stresses, traumas and ecological distress. This is achieved by harnessing your inner creative power and joining this with your favourite singer or songwriter. I present the Story Lyrics Activist and Resilience Project.

...From this inspiration you are taken on a journey

...Scientific research has demonstrated that writing is one method of resilience against issues that can sometimes overwhelm the brain. For those that have never embarked on that journey, putting pen to paper will set your free.

...Writing is one of the de-stressors from the thoughts and adversity in your mind and life,

...By entering your thoughts into your book can be one of your resilience methods for 2020.

...Writing your thoughts down on paper can provide you with a sense of hope and purpose.

...Remember the pen is mightier than the sword. If you can become an Activist through your writing you could help the three main causes in this book.

...Story Lyrics is founded on the principal of wellness attainment. You're happy moments, your stress, your nightmares, your concerns, your good and bad thoughts, your feelings and your existence can be documented by yourself in writing....Getting it all out of your mind to let your brain be at ease... to provide your brain room for fresh and positive thoughts. This process allows you to see things for what they really are. Writing could help set you free.

Story Lyrics has one pillar and

Three main causes

Pillar: That every person (including our planet) should live in true and pure equality, no discrimination, no borders, and every person is free from emotional or physical harm and abuse. A world where every person is equal to the core.

On your deathbed wealth, fame and power will remain, you can't take it with you. But kindness and goodness towards your fellow humans will go with you in perpetuity and on your next journey within the universe. This will be your only judgement on departing earth.

The Three Foundations:

1) Mental Health (Depression, Suicide and stress to name a few)

2) Missing, Abducted, Abused & Trafficked Children and Adults

3) Climate protection

Some of our websites for help

1) **DontJump.ie** established as a tool to help support people contemplating suicide by providing talks and news about different options or pathways towards staying alive.

2) **MissingInParis.com** developed as a result of a true story and it grew into a plan of action so that every person on earth can help stop this criminalised billion dollar industry and more importantly find our missing children and adults. The book and website also reviews Adverse Childhood Experiences and how they have shaped every person on earth to what they are today.

3) **StoryLyrics.com** developed as a pathway to Resilience by helping alleviate stress, anxiety and mental health problems by writing your story from the lyrics of your favourite artist.

About the Author

Dave holds a degree in Psychology and Business including a diploma in Adverse Childhood experiences. He is actively involved within the three pillars of his books. He has worked within climate adaptation, Mitigation planning and takes climate change seriously. Currently Dave is a mental health advocate and Environmental and sustainability researcher. He has carried out research and worked within the climate emergency domain over many years and has worked towards achieving sustainability within the hospitality industry. He is passionate about the seriousness of the climate emergency and asks that every person do their bit to halt Climate change.

Dave acknowledges that he is in the same conundrum as billions of other people in their personal efforts to halt climate change. He firmly believes that Governments and Politician's must be the leaders and make changes suitable for our future generation, our children, and to do it now. Governments should halt fossil fuel production, and Invest heavily in research and innovation towards sustainable transportation and energy. That technology is currently available and needs to be rolled out urgently and on a massive scale, and without profiteering.

Electric vehicles are available but the affordability cost of these is bleak for the majority of people. As such industry and Governments need to be proactive and make these affordable for everyone. Massive innovation into research re advancing the electric sustainability of aircraft is needed urgently. People need to quickly adapt to a greener and sustainable lifestyle. Changing the layout of cities to become 'smarter' with less dependence on transportation, and with a 100% switch to green sustainable energy, these are a few of the many ways ahead to a cleaner and brighter future for humanity.

MENTAL HEALTH is important for human growth, and any adversities that you endured as a child and growing up holds the key to open a door in your mind that could help heal you. Go to Dave's website missinginparis.com and do an adapted ACE (Adverse Childhood Experiences) survey.

MISSING CHILDREN and ADULTS is held dearly to Dave's heart. He was involved with searching for a missing teenager which dramatically changed his outlook in life. You can read about his experience in the book "Missing in Paris" Dave continues to look for other missing children and adults in all of his travels and he believes that everyone can do the same. Together we can all make a difference and reunite a lost one with their family and friends.

They fill the news with reports of fake and doctored images of models to creative artists to singer's songs being auto-changed. The author believes that your true nature and purity of being a person and artist has been removed and exchanged as a necessity of unnatural purity. His writing has no "auto-tune" it flows the way I write it, therefore you may come across English that does not meet the requirements of "proper grammar." He makes no apologies, the concept behind Dave's Story Lyrics brand is to get everyone writing, to free themselves from negative or inactive thoughts and replace them with positive steps that can enhance their own and others life's.

As such Dave encourages everyone to write regardless of their education or perceived correct use of grammar. Most books that are released are edited and re-edited and puffed up for glorification beyond the capabilities of one person to do. This is a barrier, don't let it be a barrier for you. JUST WRITE.

The need for perfection is a barrier to true and real creativity, too many artists hide behind a mirage of perfection to give them an identity that is fake.

There are too many people wanting to correct your grammar etc. To many critics that make you feel ashamed of yourself or what you do. But rise above them and do it, write!

You are perfect, you do not need the acclaim from others to prove that. You are perfect.

So as Dave says:

- **Look** for missing people on your travels
- **Fight** to end adversity for children and adults
- **Get** Writing
- **Become** a Climate Activist
- **Help** reduce mental health issues
- **Put** Health before wealth
- **Believe** in yourself
- **And** campaign for freedom and equality for every person in the world. We all bleed the same blood. Borders need to be removed to allow our world to finally unite.

Exiting a Lockdown

Draw a line under the world's monetary loss and strip billionaires of such obscene riches.

The financial drain on the world's economy will be validated as countries exit from their lockdowns. They have reported from many sources that we could face a financial depression not seen before. I believe that the world needs to draw a line under their monetary loss. I believe that they should not be allowed to pass this debt onto the ordinary people via taxes and any other method of monetary extraction from ordinary people. I believe that the current economic model has run its course and has seen its days for any future existence.

Current pension funds could be radically reduced in value, as share prices have dropped considerably. Will Governments help the elderly with their pension funds?

Moreover, I fully believe that the time to strip billionaires from their money and assets is now. We need to demonstrate to the little people of the world that billionaire wealth is obscene. There are approximately 2,825 billionaires around the world. There is no chance that all of the population could achieve this sickening accumulation of wealth as a normality. There are 7.8 billion people in the world and that number is growing dramatically each year. Therefore, the freedom of any pro capitalism claim is misleading and corrupt at the highest degree. It is a falsehood designed for the rich to get richer at the expenses of all the little people. Being a billionaire and keeping that wealth is no aspiration to be proud of. It is not an accomplishment to be proud of. Unless your billionaire plan is to use that wealth to fund poverty, homelessness and inequality in its totality.

The USA has a billionaire at the helm of its nation. A billionaire that believes he is better than every other person on earth. A billionaire that believes he can do and say what he wants and get away with it. People in his administration agree with him in the fear of losing their job. Again money comes first. This needs to be transformed to Health before wealth. And now in 2020, we saw Donald Trump attempting to become a dictator, a person who believes that he can thwart the democracy of the USA in order to remain in power. Donald Trump has incited violence and yet he still remains free. If that was you, you would be in jail.

Springboard for change and financial implications of an exit

The current pandemic is providing an opportunistic springboard for change, a change that will help every person in the world. If we continue to let the Trumps, and other rich, and Politian's that are motivated via donations and a claim to be rich and famous then we are doomed as a world. We need to end this hierarch that only represents an extreme minority of the world's population.

So this brings us to how do we exit a lockdown? If finance comes first, then the health of all nations are still at risk. If we follow any of the world's economic models of exit, then the coronavirus will become another "flu, cancer, etc." and any subsequent coronavirus death will join all other viruses and diseases and be known as collateral damage.

I believe that any financial based model on exiting a lockdown is inherently flawed as deaths will be justified for the glory of the masses. Where in reality it is only for the glory of the rich and not for the masses of people. Current financial models are not designed for the mass of people. Some countries do not take into account welfare for their people and other countries models include some form of welfare. However, financial models are designed so that businesses and their owners can continue to make obscene profits at the expenses of other people's deaths by justifying their actions via jobs. Jobs = taxes = Government happiness, again all at the expense of the little people and, all while the rich get richer. Any person who then becomes a multi-millionaire or billionaire defiantly has paid nowhere near their fair share in taxes.

Even the legal system is corrupt, they force legality upon you. And if you have the money, then you can receive a better legal defence. For those that cannot get legal aid, companies take advantage of this situation. And even if you get legal aid, you don't receive what multimillionaires can afford. They force justice and legalities upon all of us, therefore this must be equal, and no longer can you accept businesses or rich individuals being represented by a "better legal team" than that of the person or business with little or no money. The justice system needs to be overhauled to provide an equal legal right and certainly not defined by how rich you are or how and if you can afford a legal representation.

Now that last paragraph might seem like a rambling, but in actual fact the legality of exiting a lockdown must be talked about. Unscrupulous businesses and the wealthy will use the legal framework to get their own ends from any exit. After all, they can afford a legal team with far better knowledge and resources than you could ever dream of. This is a direct and legal manipulation of the legal right for every person to have equal representation.

Under the current legislation the little people do not have equal representation. Little people have to pay for any legal action or legal defence out of our own pockets. The rich will beat your hands down most times. So much so that they keep you from the court rooms because of not being able to afford it. Now that isn't fair at all. Therefore, do you expect any exit from a lockdown to be in your best interests? Or will be it for the best interest of the financial economy and the wealth or rich?

Regardless of any exit plan, Covid-19 is not disappearing any time soon. In fact the medical authorities believe it could become an annual event.

Look at transportation and an alternative model of working from home

Before the exit let's look at transportation, how will that work? Let's take aeroplanes, their air system is recycling the same air around the aircraft. Wearing a mask will have little impact, you will still breathe the air that everyone else is exhaling. Ok, so next point there can be no full flights as before, right? I think we can all agree to limit deaths from this virus but we must continue to have some social distancing and cleanliness plan, right? If aircraft now fly with ¼ or ½ full flights what impact will this have on climate change reduction plans? We cannot allow the rich to be the only ones who can travel by air that cannot be allowed by the people, full stop.

Buses, trains, underground trains, taxis, boats and cruise ships. Wow, what a dilemma, to practice social distancing on these forms of transportation would be a nightmare. Have you ever travelled on London's underground? I have frequently and stood sardine packed while sniffing the arm pits of the passengers next to me on all sides. This can no longer occur under the new normal, can it? Therefore all forms of transportation must have a reduced capacity to maintain a reasonable social distance, right? Again what about the damage of this to climate change?

We cannot under any circumstance exit a lockdown without regard for Climate Change and Peoples Health and Welfare. We cannot allow our Governments and legal system to exit by saying fuck you to climate change and people's health. This cannot be an exit to put pounds or dollars or whatever into the pockets of the rich.

Pubs, restaurants, cinemas, sports gatherings, entertainment gatherings etc. How will this work? Again you cannot have full gatherings without putting people's health at risk. Socialising, we all miss, being trapped in our own homes with some outdoor exercising is having a drastic effect on everyone. So much so that Tiktok and other social media platforms have seen many people go nuts with their social media posts. Will people go back to their old ways and believe that they are invincible and continue to be members of the "big crowd"?

Office workers and the manufacturing line. Many of these people work in close proximity of each other, how will this work on the lockdown exit. Is it business as normal? Or will working from home and reduced numbers of staff in an office or production line become the norm, I think it should? Working from home could be an ideal climate friendly thing to do. Less travel = less pollution. Less building size = more space for greenery and co2 sinks.

Early warning virus system

Will countries develop an early warning system to detect cases of this and other viruses? Northern Ireland have developed an app that will highlight if you have come near a person who carries coronavirus. But that app will be judged only by the number of people who have been tested and have tested positive. It will not include the many people who have caught the virus and have displayed none of the symptoms, and they will continue to move freely while infecting others.

Another consideration about maintaining 2 metres apart. You are waiting in a line to enter a shop or you are out walking. The wind is around 5 mph. A person coughs or sneezes without shielding the droplet exhalation. Those droplets travel over 2 metres. An entire line of people have now come into contact with that persons droplets. If that person is an unknown carrier, then many are now at risk.

Any exit plan, must ensure a restriction to the number of people in confined spaces, especially indoors. But it must also ensure that they maintain a constant cleanliness on a regular basis, indoors and outdoors.

Virus Testing

The speed at which some countries carried out testing was "crap." Despite warnings from the past, Governments around the world are spending more on weapons than halting the spreading of a virus epidemic, as such no plan of action was initially made. Which is extremely strange under the circumstance of people being murdered by germ warfare and the possibility of other countries using germ/virus warfare?

While the UK have been carrying out tests on a new "virus protection" scheme with human as the Guinee pigs, we are still years away from any deployment if they follow normal Government guidelines on the release of a new vaccine. Unless the financial need becomes the overwhelming decision to release this protection sooner. What I can say is: There are cancer treatments that have been withheld while awaiting years of trials, so people that are dying from cancer die. You would have thought these people could be the Guinee pig for a drug that might save their life, right? So for Governments too fast track the coronavirus vaccine would show that Governments are more concerned with a financial economy than anything else.

Testing, was a crux of stopping the spread and hence deaths from this virus. Therefore, testing should form a huge role on any countries exit and subsequent reduction in new cases and deaths.

What did China do with their exit from lockdown?

An extract from the Lancet, describes how China are being more open than many other countries. *"Although, in the past, China has been criticised for a lack of transparency related to epidemiological surveillance data, this rapid openness goes beyond what most countries are doing today... Rapid analyses, including computational modelling efforts, are vital to assist decision makers in these uncharted waters; however, these analyses are only as good as their data. Our daily understanding of the pandemic is based on the number of confirmed cases reported (e.g., WHO daily reports and online dashboards), which can only be interpreted with an understanding of who is being tested (e.g., only severe cases) and laboratory capacity."* Source April 02, 2020DOI: https://doi.org/10.1016/S1473-3099(20)30264-4

So from the statement above we can see that any exit will be only as good as the data being received. Therefore, the control point would be the number of people being tested. Test the entire population of the world and we are getting nearer to an accurate model worthy of exit dissemination.

Olympic medals

If we look at lockdowns of the world as an Olympic game, then China gets Gold medal, Italy gets Silver medal…USA gets a debunk and an IDIOT-1 medal for their lack of initial and subsequent concern. But what would you expect from a USA president that has cut billions of dollars from stopping climate change?

IDIOT-1 President Trump (2020): *"No one knew that there would be a pandemic or epidemic of this proportion."* Donald Trump.

President Obama [2014 – just over 5 and a half years ago]: *"There may and likely will come a time in which we have both an airborne disease that is deadly. And In order for us to deal with that affectively we have to put in place an infrastructure not just here at home, but globally that allows us to see it quickly and isolate quickly and respond to it quickly. So then if and when a new strain of flu like the Spanish flu props up 5 years from now or a decade from now we have made the investment and we are further along to be able to catch it. It is a smart investment for us to make. Not just insurance, it is knowing that down the road we will continue to have problems like this, particularly in a globalised world."* Barack Obama

While coronavirus is not known to be airborne, what Obama has stated has been said by the WHO and many other scientific researchers frequently in the past regarding airborne virus and transmittable viruses when in contact with another person.

Yet the current president of the USA said that coronavirus took us all by surprise. It was no surprise, it was a certainty that something like this would occur. Especially with increasing populations. What I'm surprised at, is with the emergence and threat of bio-warfare that the worlds Governments have not developed a model and system of curbing and limiting any such virus exposure. If they had, then the number of infections and deaths via coronavirus would have been decimated.

What is blatantly obvious with the USA president Donald Trump, he takes no responsibility at all for anything? Zero responsibility, it is always someone else's fault.

If you look at the Apprentice, Lord Sugar is continually firing apprentices for their lack of accepting responsibility. Perhaps Mr Trump should take a leaf from his own TV series that he originally created. Start accepting fucking responsibility Mr President.

I'm sure that Trump and his son-in-law advisors businesses will not be suffering as much as every other USA business. I'm further convinced that some Whitehouse weasels have come up with a plan that will shield Trump and his business empires from failure while making it look like we are helping all businesses, it what's called "legal tape and loopholes."

Some difficulties of an exit

The following document outlines some difficulties in an exit from a lockdown: The author further states that this first round will not be enough to halt this pandemic.

"The aim of these measures, such as social distancing, is not to bring the number of people infected down to zero, Leung said; "that is not possible." Rather, they are an effort to protect older people, who have a much higher risk of becoming infected and dying, as well as to keep health-care systems functioning. "No country, no population, no city can be spared from COVID-19," said Leung, who is advising the Hong Kong Government on its response to the virus. "The big question is, how do you make sure that you do not overwhelm societal functions? How do you make sure that your hospital system does not collapse? How do you make sure that there are enough ICU beds and ventilators for those who need them? How do you make sure that you can minimize the morbidity and mortality burden on your population while protecting the economy and the livelihood of the people on a sustainable basis? These are the big questions that any society would have to grapple

with and have been grappling with."

https://www.theatlantic.com/international/archive/2020/03/lockdowns-hong-kong-china-coronavirus/608932/ Timothy McLaughlin on 28/3/2020

As established above it becomes a trade-off, a balance of acceptable deaths vs sustaining a countries economy. Therefore, I believe that any exit from a lockdown will enviable hold consequences. But I ask you one question, if you knew that your child would die if the lockdown ended for purely financial reasons, would you accept that your child's death was worthy of collateral damage for the good of others wealth creation, would you accept that?

We have a report in the Guardian newspaper claiming that they cannot stop any lockdown until we have found a vaccine to counteract this virus. Well for all those that have had a loved one die from cancer when there was a possible proven drug that had not finished its testing but was showing a cure rate, then I would say fuck you for not providing this drug. So in a nutshell because the world has gone into lockdown the financial implications dictate that it is fast forwarded past the normal time for testing etc. and release it as soon as. Is this morally just, when we have let millions die from cancer and AIDS because of a lack to release vaccines sooner than later?

The report by Sarah Boseley further states, *"China's aggressive controls over daily life have brought the first wave of Covid-19 to an end, say researchers based in Hong Kong. But the danger of a second wave is very real."*

Well great for China. Did you hear that Mr Trump, and some other world leaders? China's quick action and not letting people do what they want was directly responsible for keeping their death toll at a minimum (4,633). Whereas here in the UK (over 33,614 deaths), USA (86,937 deaths) and in many other countries, the attitude was, "that's a restriction to our freedom of rights," these are the comments from people who I can only explain as ignoramuses, people with little regard for other people safety. (Data as at 15th May 2020)

No true lockdown

Even today, there is no true lockdown in the UK, people are still manipulating the rules to do what they want. I just seen six lads from different families walk past my house all within inches of each with some cans of beer, going for a bevy by the riverfront. I have heard that some pubs around the country are having a lock-in. Mass gatherings for funerals, social gatherings etc. Are these people for real? These people might not know that they are carriers of the virus. These are the people who are probably responsible for spreading the virus. These are the people who think they can do what they want while the rest of us obey the rules.

The news is filled with people coming within close contact of each other. Instead of one person doing the essential shopping, it's a couples outing. It's a fucking day out, not a lockdown. I just came back from doing the shopping on my own as usual. Yet the outdoor shopping area that I went to was full people not practising social distancing, it was an evening out.

Now that is the difference between China and us. That's why China's death toll is massively less than ours. But fuck that, why would anyone put themselves out to help save someone else's life, right? After all, we live in the free world, right? What a pile of shite, the people with no regard to safety measures are the ones responsible for spreading and ultimately killing people.

Speed of Lockdowns

Because of the dramatic number of deaths Italy was one of the first to go into a lockdown after China. Presumably they will be one of the first to attempt an exit from lockdown. While the world wants to move on and break free, it needs to be completed in a controlled manner with people's health and welfare coming first.

They have reported that Italy's Prime Minister Giuseppe Conte is seeking scientific advice on how best to exit when the time is ready. This is the same with many other countries. But how countries will exit will based on their best economic model. This is wrong and morally unjust. While people want to get back to work to earn a living. I believe that a humanistic model would ensure that every person on earth has the right to life, equality, a home, food and an infrastructure and this should replace the current financial models. But unfortunately a humanistic model cannot justify 2,153 billionaires (as per Forbes November 2019) or multi-millionaires that exists in our world today. But what it can have is a society where people care for each other and health comes before wealth accumulation.

It has been further stated by many that the exit from lockdown must be a gradual process of bringing normality back on line, and not by a total end to the lockdown. Again the cases and deaths within a country or particular area of a country will be the main contributing factor in determining if a country is reducing its coronavirus infections and deaths.

Travel virus testing

Should people be stopped from travelling, even if they are diagnosed with a cold or flu? Should travel insurance companies be forced to ensure that people are covered for any possibly delay in travel because of a virus or flu? I think so.

Travel will place an enormous weight on all efforts to contain the virus within your country. Testing will need to be done at airports and transportation hubs before we consider any travel. Are countries at that stage yet and do they have enough resources to meet the demands for travel? Fewer people than normal should only be admitted to airports and onward transportation.

When will tourists come back on line? Holiday makers seeking sun, partygoers seeking fun and a busy night life in a foreign country. Until we have a vaccine or a total control over the virus any attempt to induce a tourist trade as before would be reckless of any country or person to do. Under a financial model what about these business how long will Governments support them? What about their employees are Governments going to continue supporting them to?

School Children

School children cannot return to their normal high numbers of children per classroom. What implication and cost will this put on the shoulders of those with educational decisions and their corresponding budgets? Classrooms and schools should be less than ½ full from now on from an exit.

With a phased exit, decisions on what businesses may open first and to what extend can they reopen. For example, we cannot have production lines with people right next to each other, like battery hens.

Animals to should have some form of social distancing

Inhumane animal living conditions, like battery hens for mass production must cease. Most coronavirus and other virus affecting animals and then humans have been directly due to some contamination of food sources directly because of close proximity of animals and the way these animals are kept and butchered. In a nutshell how would you feel if you were trapped in a compact room with 100 other people, before they massacred you?

Evidence has also highlighted that the areas were few cases have occurred or where the cases and deaths are reducing is directly because of the method of their lockdown and hence containment of the virus.

Social and economic implications

Italy has further warned that any exit could have implications for many people on both for social and economic reasons. With any phased exit café's, restaurants and other small businesses in relation to tourism could take up to an extra three months to reopen. And even then, the rest of the world will probably not be able to travel as tourists or on business as they did before coronavirus reared its ugly head.

It has been declared that bars and nightclubs will be the last to reopen in Italy. I can hear the Irish saying "Like fuck it will be."

Regardless the world will face a financial deficit that will take 2 to 5 years if not more to recover from. The people should not have to pay this price. If we take the Trillions from the billionaires, then that should cover most of it. The time for nationalisation of large industries is now. We can no longer allow the minority to control and decide for the majority, while the rich defecate themselves in wealth over that of humanity.

An exit has a multitude of decisions

As you can see any exit plan has a multitude of decisions to be prepared, some of which could have a dramatic impact on our next future pandemic, that being climate change. If we don't do the right thing here and now, then your children will face an epidemic that will make the total world deaths of any virus look minuscule. Climate change is happening here and right now, the fact that you won't face the totality of its consequences now, gives you a false sense of guard. But if you do nothing now and let others away from doing nothing towards halting climate cancer, then you have sealed the fate for your children and their children, as such don't expect any perceived god to welcome you with open arms.

Ireland has just release its roadmap to a phased exit from our worldwide pandemic. They have suggested 5 phases, 1st phase beginning on 18th May 2020 and phase 5 on 10th of August 2020. All phases will depend on how well the containment of the virus goes. Ireland as of 2nd May 2020 has had 20,833 cases and 1,265 deaths. They also went into a lockdown prior to the UK, which was a bit concerning as the north of Ireland came under UK rules and regulations. It will be interesting to see what will occur on the island of Ireland as far as the lockdown and the pandemic exit is concerned. There needs to be a unilateral agreement between Stormont, UK and Irish Governments.

While many of the exit plans will be difficult to monitor, such as when in someone's home you have to wear a face mask, who will enforce this? While they are playing the card of hope and trust. There will be people in the community who will sadly disregard these rules and put other people's lives at risk.

The Irish phased website can be found at:

https://www.gov.ie/en/press-release/e5e599-Government-publishes-roadmap-to-ease-covid-19-restrictions-and-reope/

On the 1st of May 2020, Boris Johnson announced that the UK is past its peak cases and deaths. He suggested that the country "can now see the sunlight." He has also stated that it's too early yet to lift restrictions, but in the coming week he will set out plans for "kick-starting the economy."

With these comments in mind, I hope that the Tory Government remember two things, first, the impact of their proposals and plans on climate change and the how they plan to help the people?

As of the 2nd May 2020, the UK has had 182,260 cases and 28,131 deaths.

All exits must include common sense

All exist from any countries lockdown will signify the first wave, but really do we want a second wave of cases and deaths? Measures need to be put in place to stop any recurring infections. A vaccine and common sense should be present within any decisions.

- It is common sense not to put your hand in a fire.
- It's common sense to wash your hands regularly.
- It's common sense to practice social distancing
- Its common sense that people's Health should come before

wealth.

- It's common sense that we can no longer have masses of people in the one area for the foreseeable future
- It is common sense that there is no planet B to live on.
- It is common sense that one piece of shit in a bath pollutes all the water.
- It is common sense that every tonne of co2, methane etc. that we pour into our atmosphere pollutes the entire world
- It is common sense that melting ice sheets and glaziers will raise sea levels which reduces land mass. Plus a lot more.
- It is common sense that we should help to end poverty, homelessness, inequality and oppression.
- It is common sense that most cancer deaths is due to pollution by fossil fuels etc.
- It is common sense that smokers can die with cancer
- It is common sense to have an adequate exit plan and roadmap that will safeguard the population of the world
- Unfortunately, It's common sense that our leaders lack

Testing and Re-testing

- The biggest piece of common sense. We should have full scale testing available.
- Testing before someone travels to another country. Testing when a person arrives into a country. Including staff involved with transportation of food and goods between other countries.
- Testing when a person enters a hospital or doctors. Testing helps stop the virus from spreading to others, which reduces the number of infections and deaths.

Conclusion and roadmap in a nutshell

I have always been fascinated by the term "in a nutshell." I was 11 years old, and we went on a trip called "Norway in a nutshell," since then I can't get that term or usage out of my mind.

The only feasible way out of a pandemic lockdown can only be when the number of cases and deaths have reduced drastically. I'm avoiding saying to an acceptable level for the simple reason that would accommodate any other deaths as acceptable collateral damage. No deaths should be accredited as collateral damage to aid a financial model of an economy. If any leader said that they would accept the death of their loved one as collateral damage then they would be one of the following. a) A lying bar Stewart or b) An inconsiderate Punt

Ok, so we enter phase one of any exit. We don't want a second lockdown or second phase. Therefore, essential businesses and productions can come on line again first on a larger scale as of the past but still the need to maintain social distancing and practising safe cleaning and hygiene rules.

[**As of December 2020**, there have been several lockdowns of various degrees, circuit breaker lockdowns, tier 1, 2 and 3 lockdowns. We have become a world of new terminology towards inventing new names and logic for the realms of lockdowns and continued lockdowns. In the current nine months of the pandemic, this displays a total lack of leadership and knowledge on the best ways forward to exit a pandemic. This has further cost countries horrendous cost in lives lost and has been a major burden on world economies. And the cost of jobs and income reduction for many people. This has led to a dramatic increase in poverty and to the number of vulnerable people around the world.]

A return to work for office workers on a phased rollout. Meaning we cannot have full offices, so perhaps people rotate their shifts to stop overcrowding, while maintaining a good cleaning and disinfectant routine. This principal would have to apply to all business, schools, sports centres, swimming pools etc. Though hygienic and safe distancing would need to be maintained at all times and well into the future. In fact I believe that it should become the standard.

Restaurants and cafes could offer takeaways, the problem with sitting in, you may have a table full of people, which under a first phases roll out could help transmit the virus again. This situation also fuels a false sense of security where people actively forget about the problem and become closer than what would be liked. The wearing of masks for customers in these type of places would be fraught with problems. How could you eat or drink? However, I would suggest that floor staff and food preparation staff should wear masks at all times.

Bars and other social places

Bars, pubs and night clubs, sports and entertainment fixtures well that's a whole different ball game, how can you practice social distance in these types of businesses or events? "Excuse me", as you shout to the person 2 metres away, "would you like to dance?" then maintaining a safe distance apart? I believe that because of the complexities of restricting numbers these types of business should be the last to reopen. Doing so has a further drawback for the tourism trade. Going to bars, pubs, clubs and restaurants or a sporting event is what most people do when they go on a holiday or a night out at their local hubs. Again I would suggest that all staff wear face masks.

Transportation and Airlines

Travelling on transportation needs to be controlled to limit the number of people who can travel at once. At no time should the rich be able to travel before anyone else, in other words no price hiking should be used to reduce anyone's travelling ability. Being and staff on transportation could wear masks.

It is not rocket science to considerate the impact on airlines. In Europe we could see several airlines going into receivership. It has been reported that there are over 110 airlines in Europe, therefore it would be reasonable to predict that many will either be amalgamated with other airlines or go bust. The UK Government did not stand by Flybe, they went into receivership in the early days the pandemic. Will countries stand by other airlines financially?

I believe that Governments will be selective in which airlines they will try to save. For example after restrictions are lifted and countries begin to exit the lock-down, will people want to travel as before? Would you want to be packed into a full flight and a full airport? Thus, why would Governments bail out airlines that will be a drain on the economy, there is only so much help that Governments can provide under an economic model? Then the people are the ones that suffer via higher taxes.

One thing for sure, we cannot allow prices to be fixed so that the rich or wealth have an upper hand to that of the people. Meaning they will not fly before anyone else. Nor should their wealth provide any travel incentive over the little people.

After lock-down has ended?

- Will you get on a full bus?

- Will you get on a full train?

- Will you get on a full flight?

- Will you go into a full office?

- Will you attend a full sports fixture?

- Will you attend a full concert?

- Will you enter a full shop?

- Will you wear a mask or not?

- Will you go to a beach packed by people?

- Will you stay in a full hotel?

- Will you go to a full restaurant?

- Will you go into a packed pub?

- Will you work in a full production line?

- Will you ....?

If your answer to the above is "no," then the implications could be profound. Fewer people implies higher costs and less income for businesses and workers.

Under the circumstances companies, shareholders and owners should not be able to profiteer. We must see an end to billionaires, multi-millionaires and obscene company profits.

When the attacks on the twin towers occurred in New York, people were afraid to travel for a while in the USA, however after around 6 to 9 months the market soon bounced back when faith was restored. The coronavirus has worldwide implications that could take the travel industry a lot longer to bounce back from. The fear of close people proximity needs to be addressed.

Countries economic models should be ratified, amended and made as a model for the people and not only to increase the ladder of the rich.

People will concerned about their jobs and hence income. What is to happen to people who lose their job because of redundancies and bankruptcy?

The exit from any lockdown must include all of the above to arrive at a decision for a plan of action and subsequent roadmap that will benefit the masses of people rather than the few.

Masks, gloves or not?

People need a total clarification by Governments, scientific and health officials on the practicality and effectiveness of wearing a mask and gloves. At present there are many conflicting stories on "should" the public wear masks or gloves? There is even news of mandatory wearing of masks when lock-down has ended. If that is the plan after exit why has it not been implemented since day one of the lockdown?

Governments and business first words is "Economy"

Another startling fact on all countries exit plans is the first words used by your leaders, "Economy." The economy is coming first from the mouths of leaders in most conversations or speeches. Health before wealth and economy should come first at all times. But sadly this is obviously not the case. Climate change plans appear to be last on their list. You would have thought for one second that because of this virus, the world leaders would open their eyes to what is occurring around the world. Such panic over a virus that has killed a hell of a lot less than the Spanish flu. Yet Climate change will make the coronavirus pandemic a walk in the park for future generations.

Climate change needs a roadmap to

If the world leaders do not acknowledge and immediately forget about the economy and put the welfare of the world's population and earth itself foremost, then they have fucked the future for your children and their children.

The time is now to create a climate change roadmap and exit plan, to remove the world from fossil fuel emissions, pollutions, poverty and inequality. If our leaders learn one thing from the coronavirus lockdown, they should learn and understand that this is only the beginning for both unknown viruses and climate change. Climate change will be responsible for introducing many new viruses via the destruction that the developing world is doing to our world's environment.

The only correct way forward is now, and it's now that our leaders need to be committed to ending climate change with tough legislations and nationalisation of many industries. We can no longer allow the wealthier to come wealthier at the expenses of all the little people of the world, that's 7.8 billion of us.

I ask a simple question, how can any of the 2,153 billionaires of the world sleep at night knowing that their wealth could end a lot of human suffering?

You can see that this pandemic has reshaped society during the lockdowns. How long will it be before people decide to screw that and go back to how it was before? But doing that will put everyone's life at risk and will make a mockery for all future pandemics.

The first exit from a worldwide pandemic will be attempted on a country to country bases. Travel from country to country should only be for essential services and foods and goods. I would expect universal individual travel to be delayed until all countries are back on line. It would be irresponsible for any country to allow masses of other people in and out of its country until the virus cases and deaths have been stabilised between member countries.

In the meantime Governments must ensure that every person are being looked after emotionally, socially and financially, including helping others in developing countries.

Sports fixtures, the rich and famous

What could be considered alarming is the football associations are already talking about travelling to other countries that have either contained the virus or it hasn't got there yet, with the aim to complete their league without their fans in presence, more of an online televised event? I'm sure many fans would love that idea.

However, if they are permitted to compete in sports then I and millions of others demand our right to visit our families and friends. Is it money that speaks, or the fact that they have a legal team and we don't? Or what?

It's one rule for all, no exceptions, the fact that the EU leagues have fancy lawyers and loads of dosh, will not derail us from the fact, if they can travel then so can we.

We cannot allow the rich to travel at the expenses of the little people. Nor will they use the excuse that it could help people socially. Being allowed to visit family and friends in other countries is way more important than sports or whatever.

The football associations and any other sporting organisation can wait like everyone else before they jet around the world. And that applies to everyone, singers, artists, etc. The ordinary person will travel first before that of the rich and famous.

The rich getting their lawyers involved

In a matter of days since Ireland have released their roadmap for exiting, business have got their lawyers involved to try and reduce the time before they can re-open. Licensed bars and pubs want to re-open before August. Can you imagine sitting in a pub while practising social distancing then some drunk comes staggering over to your table?

Socially acceptable ideas

A restaurant in the Netherlands came up with a splendid idea and deployed greenhouses suitable for 2 people by the edge of the canal. Romantic, Social and safe. Providing that they change the table cloths, wipe down the seating and the glass panel within the greenhouse, now that's the risk assessment done. And the charges for food is not hiked up. For that would not be acceptable by any means. Again the rich cannot be permitted to leave the ordinary person behind.

Climate Change

In several announcements Boris Johnson and other world leaders have said that they will reduce the lockdown on advice taken from scientific advisors. Impressive stuff, yet they have totally ignored climate change scientific advice. The reason being, taking such advice will cause a lot of upheaval on our current day-to-day routines. It would cost many trillions of pounds, dollars, yen etc. to sort the problem out. So our Governments of the world drag their feet, while our earth perishes.

Climate change will be a pandemic of magnitude proportions that cannot and will not be straightforwardly fixed as is the COVID-19 outbreak.

If you value your children and their children's future then you must stand up and become an activist for climate change today, and with action today. You need to make your Governments submit to fixing earth now. If they will not be the leaders, then we need to take that leadership from them and do it ourselves.

Last words and remembrance

The percentage based figures below are deaths divided by number of cases. Therefore the death rate is based on that resolve.

As of 26th December 2020, worldwide there have been 80,552,867 cases and 1,762.920 deaths from coronavirus. That represents 2.2% of people tested positive will die. Big difference percentage based on those outlined below. Why? Is it that the vulnerable are better protected? Or are Governments around the world providing false figures? Or ?

As of 2nd May 2020, worldwide there have been 3,456,231 cases and 243,024 deaths from coronavirus. That represents 7% of people tested positive will die.

As at 5th May 2020, worldwide there have been 3,665,418 cases and 252,950 deaths from coronavirus. That represents 6.9% of people tested positive will die.

As at 7th May 2020, worldwide there have been 3,870,751 cases and 267,761 deaths from coronavirus. That represents 6.9% of people tested positive will die.

As at 20th May 2020, worldwide there have been 5,018,657 cases and 325,673 deaths from coronavirus. That represents 6.5% of people tested positive will die.

As at 17th December 2020, worldwide there have been 75,204,485 cases and 1,666,636 deaths from coronavirus. That represents 2, 2% of people tested positive will die

As you can see the death percentage rates are reducing the more people are being tested and social distancing and hygienic measures are applied.

In eighteen days there was an increase of 1,562,426 cases and an increase of 82,649 deaths around the world.

Some countries cases and deaths are reducing while other countries are beginning to be infected. With any exit plan, they must factor the wave effect in. The wave effect is when cases and deaths are at the peak height of the wave, the wave then falls while cases and deaths reduce. Moreover, waves always rise again, so a proper plan of action and roadmap needs to be put in place to calm the wave.

I don't believe that we should allow any% of deaths due to coronavirus to be recognised as collateral damage now or in the future. What do you think? I believe that we must have a new economic model that suits every person on earth, so when any other pandemic begins it should be no big deal shutting up shop.

We also need a plan of action for the 272 million migrants stranded around the world. Who will help them?

Let's take a moment to remember all those that have died on earth. While their current existence on earth has sadly ended, their family, friends, colleagues and neighbours will remember them. In a world with many religions, faiths, gods and atheist belief's, may your own belief be with you in these times of need.

Regarding our climate emergency, if you only remember three things, remember these:

1. Radical climate justice is required now, or the future will become your children's nightmare

2. Put Health and Equality before wealth

"Mother Earth is a source of life, and not a resource"
Chief Arvol Looking Horse

www.ingramcontent.com/pod-product-compliance
Lightning Source LLC
Chambersburg PA
CBHW062115040426

42336CB00041B/1049